JOGGING

A Guide to Successful Aerobics

Third Edition

DALE E. CAMPBELL

American Press
Boston, Massachusetts

PREFACE

Although the late 1970s and 1980s were years that indicated a significant increase in the number of individuals jogging in our country, many others were failing miserably in their attempts to attain optimum physical fitness levels. Why have so many people taken up aerobics as a form of exercising? Many men and women have approached aerobic exercising as a "cure-all" to "undo" the hazards of an unstructured and undisciplined lifestyle. In many cases, individuals start too strenuously, leaving them with a feeling of stress and without the desired outcome of optimum physical fitness. This type of unstructured approach leads to many giving up aerobics as a way of exercising.

Many people have turned to aerobics in hopes of renewed health and vitality. Man is constantly striving for a sense of control over his own destiny. This can be partially accomplished by attaining optimum physical fitness. A positive mental and physical release may also be experienced through participation in an aerobics program often leading to a more balanced and harmonious coexistence.

Accompanying this quest for an adequate aerobics program came the need to seek out pertinent contributions to the literature in this area. With the jogging boom of the 1970s, there came a large number of books onto the market dealing with that topic. Many of the books published dealing with jogging or running were virtually useless to the beginning jogger. There was a lack of creditable, well-researched literature that was appropriate for a beginning aerobics jogging program. Many sources start discussing a beginning program but quickly progress to training for road-racing and marathons. The purpose of the text is to devise a manual relevant to a beginning aerobics jogging program. For clarity in writing and ease of reading, the masculine form of pronouns is used to denote both men and women.

In chapter 1 of this new edition includes updated information from the "Healthy People 2010" report in relationship to the need for our population to be more physically active. Our culture continues to suffer the consequences of having such a sedentary lifestyle. Included in Chapter 11 is a new section dealing with over exposure to ultraviolet rays. The risk of skin cancer can be minimized greatly by the proper use of sunscreens, the wearing of proper clothing, wearing a hat, and the use of sunglasses. This edition also includes a new chapter (13) dealing with cross training. Cross-training is an excellent way in which to add variety and fun to your training program.

ACKNOWLEDGEMENTS

The author wishes to extend his appreciation to Scot Bennett and Susan Schultz for their work on the photography; Megan Smith and Josh Raymond, the two runners on the cover photo; J. Garrison, Kathy Stockin, Steven Young, and my spring semester of 1993 Jogging class for their time and patience as models; my colleagues in the physical education department for the supportive academic climate they have created at Houghton College; Dr. Guy Penny, Dr. A.H. Solomon, and Dr. Charles Babb from Middle Tennessee State University for the encouragement, guidance, and creative contributions they made; my wife Lynn, for her support and professional editing for this text; and my children Craig and Erin, may they grow to appreciate the benefits of a physically active lifestyle.

ABOUT THE AUTHOR

Dale E. Campbell did his undergraduate and graduate training at University of Nevada, Las Vegas. He completed his Doctorate at Middle Tennessee State University. Dr. Campbell is an Associate Professor of Kinesiology at Vanguard University in Costa Mesa, CA. Dr. Campbell has taught at the college level for over 20 years in both areas of physical education pedagogy and a wide variety of activity courses. He is an avid long distance runner and routinely competes at both the local and international levels in masters competition. He currently competes for Team Runners High based out of Long Beach, CA and recently won the gold medal at the World Masters Championships in the 3,000-meter Steeplechase held in Edmonton, Canada.

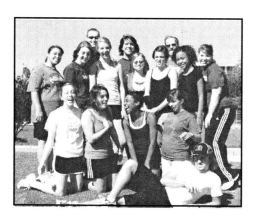

CONTENTS

xi

DEFINITION OF TERMS

Acclimatization — Adaptation to an environmental condition such as temperature or altitude.

Adipose Tissue — Tissue in which fat is stored.

Aerobic — Activity which requires the presence of oxygen to sustain.

Aerobic fitness — Maximum ability to take in, transport, and utilize oxygen.

Alveoli — Tiny air sacs in the lungs where oxygen and carbon dioxide exchange takes place.

Amino Acids — Combine to form the protein that is used to build cell walls, muscles, hormones, enzymes, and a variety of other molecules.

Anaerobic — Activity which does not require the presence of oxygen to sustain.

ATP (Adenosine Triphosphate) — High energy compound formed from oxidation of fats and carbohydrates.

Atrophy — Loss of size of muscle when not used regularly.

Blood pressure — Force of blood exerted against the walls of arteries.

Calories — Amount of heat required to raise one kilogram of water one degree centigrade.

Capillaries — Smallest blood vessels where oxygen, foods, and hormones are delivered to tissues and carbon dioxide and wastes are picked up.

Carbohydrate — Simple and complex foodstuff that is used for energy being stored in liver and muscle as glycogen with excessive amounts stored as fat.

Cardiac — Pertaining to the heart.

Cardiac output — Volume of blood pumped by the heart, determined by heart rate and stroke volume.

Cardiovascular endurance — Term used to denote aerobic fitness or maximal oxygen uptake.

Cardiovascular system — Pertains to heart and blood vessels.

Cholesterol — Fatty substance formed in blood vessels and other tissues which can lead to higher risk of heart disease.

Dehydration — Loss of essential body fluids.

Diastolic pressure — Lowest pressure exerted by blood in arteries occurring during the resting phase of the heart cycle.

Endurance — The ability to persist and resist fatigue.

Enzyme — An organic catalyst that accelerates the rate of chemical reactions.

Evaporation — Elimination of body heat when sweat vaporizes on the surface of skin.

Exercise — Term used to denote any form of physical activity involving exertion.

Fast twitch muscle fibers — Fast contracting muscle fibers that are efficient in regards to explosive power, but fatigue very rapidly.

Fat — Energy source stored for future use when excessive fat, carbohydrate, or protein is ingested.

Fatigue — Diminished work capacity, usually short of true physiological limits.

Flexibility — Range of motion through which the body is able to move.

Glucose — Energy source transported in the blood primarily essential for proper functioning of brain and nervous tissue.

Glycogen — Storage form of glucose found in liver and muscles.

Heart rate — Frequency of contraction of the heart, commonly referred to as pulse rate.

Hemoglobin — Iron compound in red blood cells that forms loose association with oxygen.

Interval training — Training method that alternates short bouts of intense effort with periods of active recuperation.

Lactic acid — Byproduct of anaerobic glycolysis.

Maximal oxygen uptake (Intake, consumption) — Most efficient method of measuring fitness in relationship to cardiorespiratory endurance.

Metabolism — Energy production and utilization processes, often mediated by enzymatic pathways.

Muscular fitness — The strength, muscular endurance, and flexibility needed to carry out daily exercising while avoiding injury.

Obesity — Excessive body fat (over 20% for men, over 30% for women).

Overload Principle — Greater load than normally experienced in training designed to specifically develop a particular function of the body.

Oxygen debt — Recovery oxygen uptake above resting requirements to replace deficit incurred during exercise.

Oxygen deficit — Lack of oxygen in early moments of exercise.

Oxygen uptake — Oxygen used in oxidative metabolism to fuel the body during exercise.

Protein — Organic compound formed from amino acids that forms muscle tissue, hormones, enzymes, etc.

Pulse — Wave that travels through the artery after each contraction of the heart.

Respiration — Intake of oxygen from atmosphere into lungs and then through the blood to the tissues, and exhalation of carbon dioxide from tissues to the atmosphere.

Slow twitch muscle fibers — Slow contracting muscle fibers that are fatigue resistant.

Stroke volume — Volume of blood pumped from ventricle during each contraction of the heart.

Systolic Pressure — Highest pressure in arteries that results from contraction of the heart.

Tendon — Tough connective tissue that connects muscle to bone.

Triglycerides — A fat consisting of three fatty acids and glycerol.

Wind chill — Cooling effect of temperature and wind.

LIFESTYLE: THE KEY TO OPTIMAL WELL-BEING   1

Humans have a distinct need to be physically active. Until recently, we had to continually search for food or had to work hard to raise the food we needed to survive.[1] However, modern society is designed so that most of us are sitting while performing our jobs, attending school, and during recreational activities such as watching TV, reading, going to the movies, etc.

According to the 1990 Government report entitled "Healthy People 2000," less than 10% of the adult population exercise at the level recommended by the 1990 objectives of the Department of Health and Human Services (exercise involving large muscle groups in dynamic movement for periods of 20 minutes or longer, three or more days per week, and which is performed at an intensity of 60% or greater of an individual's cardiorespiratory capacity).[2] The report also emphasized that more than 40% of American adults are extremely sedentary (meaning this group of adults do very little, if any, physical exercise in a typical week). Our government has since published the "Healthy People 2010" report that entails the need as a nation to improve our overall quality of health. The report deals with 28 topics relating to two primary goals:

Goal One—Increase the quality and years of healthy life and Goal Two—Eliminate health disparities in our country.[3] Certainly aerobic programs are an important component toward meeting goal one.

A national survey conducted by Lieberman Research Inc. for *Sports Illustrated* in 1986 revealed similar results to the 1990 Healthy People 2000 report.[4] Although seven out of ten respondents reported that they participated in fitness activities during the year, the average participation for the individuals surveyed amounted to 53.2 times per year, or about once a week. Only 10% of respondents reported participating four or more times per week and 27% of respondents indicated that they did not participate in physical activities during the year. The study also showed that there were more men than women participating in regular physical activity and participation declines steadily with age. The estimates for the number of joggers in our country vary from 30 to 35 million people.[5] Currently jogging ranks as the third most popular form of exercise trailing swimming and cycling respectively.

Recent research indicates that physical inactivity is a major factor in the development of coronary heart disease (CHD) for adult populations.[6] Research also indicates that children who are more physically active reduce their chances of adopting a sedentary lifestyle and developing an adult like CHD risk profile.[7] A major goal of our society must be to get people of all ages moving and becoming physically active, but, in particular, our youth. Our society must change its view that optimal health can be purchased, legislated, and delivered in the form of medical products and medical care, to a view that emphasizes that a persons health is primarily the responsibility of the individual and that the goal is prevention of disease and sickness.[8]

Aaron Wildavsky of the University of California estimates that as much as 90 percent of the difference in health among individual Americans is determined not by medical care but by factors of lifestyle—eating habits, smoking, exercise and the environment in which we live.[9] Personal lifestyle is the variable over which we have the most control. The United States Surgeon General stated it this way in his 1979 report on Health Promotion and Disease Prevention:

Collectively smoking, misuse of alcohol and other drugs, poor dietary habits, lack of regular exercise, and stress place enormous burdens on the health and well-being of many Americans today . . . Although helping people to understand the need for and to act to change detrimental lifestyles cannot be easy, the dramatic potential benefits clearly make the effort worthwhile.[10]

AVOIDING DESTRUCTIVE HABITS

Smoking

Smoking is the largest preventable cause of death in our society. The implication of smoking and trying to institute a successful aerobics program are obvious. To be successful as a jogger, it is imperative to be able to process oxygen efficiently in the circulatory system. Smoking is a tremendous detriment to this process. Most persons who smoke are well aware of the negative consequences to their well-being. The following guidelines have been developed by the American College of Sport Medicine to be useful in providing assistance to individuals who want to stop smoking:

1. Provide information on the dangers of smoking and the benefits of quitting. Emphasize that quitting smoking is probably the single most important action they can take to improve their health

2. Determine the participants willingness to quit
3. Evaluate past failures and develop new strategies
4. Put into writing a quit date and develop a specific cessation plan
5. Provide a list of programs that can provide information and support with the cessation plan
6. Follow up and provide encouragement and support
7. Prepare for relapse.[11]

The following organizations offer assistance either at no cost or materials at low cost:

"Quit for Good" Kit
Office of Cancer Communications
National Cancer Institute
Building 31, Room 10A18
Bethesda, MD 20205

Stanford Health Promotion Resource Center
1000 Welch Road
Palo Alto, CA 94304-1885
(415) 723-1000

The following national offices can supply phone numbers for local chapters.

American Lung Association
1740 Broadway
New York, NY 10019
(212) 315-8700

American Cancer Society
1599 Cliffton Road
Atlanta, GA 30329
(404) 320-3333

WEIGHT CONTROL

Excessive body fat is a risk factor for cardiovascular disease.[12] Very few people are overweight because of hormonal or other physical disorders. The vast majority of people in our society struggle with weight control problems because of too little exercise and too high of intake of calories on a daily basis. Permanent weight loss can occur only by decreasing food consumption and by increasing energy expended through physical activity. Unfortunately many in our society are convinced that fad diets and quick result diets are the best methods to lose weight. Weight reduction must be approached with an attitude of a gradual reduction. Most people would be wise to not try to reduce more than one pound per week. This would be a gradual approach that would not require drastic changes in the individuals lifestyle.

Fad diets are not long term solutions. Most people can effectively diet long term only if it means slight modification of their present diet. Drastic changes in the diet will only mean a short term change in behavior modification. The following suggestions for weight loss have been developed by the American College of Sport Medicine:

1. Gradual approach is most successful
2. Specific changes in eating habits
   a. eat only fruit for snacks
   b. reduce fried foods
   c. eat meatless meals
   d. use a small plate
   e. put down fork between bites
   f. keep a food diary
3. Review past successes and failures with weight
4. Establish realistic short and long-term goals

5. Educate yourself regarding scientific principles for effective weight loss

6. Be prepared for relapses of previous behavior

7. Continue to monitor behavior after you have lost desired pounds.[13]

DIET

We are a nation of contradictions when it comes to food. We live in a country where supermarkets are well stocked with an abundant variety of nutritious foods; yet many Americans who can afford to eat well are malnourished. Eating is associated with good times and having fun, but our society has an obsession with being slim.[14] Most of us received the basic information that we need to know about the type of diet that we should eat on a daily basis while we were in elementary school (the four basic food groups—milk products, meats, fruits and vegetables, and grain products). From these four basic food groups comes the need for a well-balanced diet containing a wide variety of foods to provide us with the seven basic categories of nutrients (proteins, carbohydrates, fats, fiber, vitamins, minerals, and water). The greatest need of most people in our society would be to cut down on the intake of sugar, sodium, and fats in the diet.[15] A knowledge of basic nutrition enables the individual to make choices in diet planning that conforms to overall wellness goals. Understanding desirable exercise and nutrition habits can help the individual make positive choices throughout the life cycle.[16]

STRESS MANAGEMENT

"Stress" is a popular term used in our society to describe everything from daily annoyances to major emotional disorders. Mental and physical health are affected by an individual's ability to avoid or adapt to stress.[17] The mind is a complex organism that has the ability to influence the individual's health either for good or for ill. The thought process can relate memories and images that make us feel good or relaxed which stimulates health. The thought process can also cause feelings of worry or fewer that are destructive to health. Obviously it's better to increase the pleasure-producing, positive thoughts and images in the mind.[18] Although jogging is not a cure-all in relationship to stress, it can be an effective way of managing stress. It would be foolish to assume that one can eliminate all stress from his/her life. The key is to effectively manage the stress that is associated with daily living patterns consistent with our society. Physical activity should be an important tool in this on-going challenge.

OSTEOPOROSIS

Osteoporosis refers to the loss of total bone mass to such an extent that the skeleton is unable to maintain its mechanical integrity. The development of this condition is a complex process influenced by a lack of calcium in the diet, sedentary lifestyle, hormonal changes (especially after menopause), and genetic factors. Normal aging causes the bones to lose mass. Women begin to lose bone mineral at about age 30 and men at approximately 50 years of age.[19] This problem is more pronounced in women than in men. Women will lose approximately .75% to 1% bone mass per year during the third decade of life. This will increase to a higher rate of 2% to 3% after menopause. Men over 50 lose about .4% per year in bone mass.[20] The total bone loss by age 70 would be approximately 25% to 30% for women, and 12% to 15% for men. Women at this age are four times more likely to break or fracture bones than are men. While continued research is needed to determine how to reverse this trend, it certainly appears that physical activity may play a key role in the maintenance of skeletal integrity.

An aerobics jogging program should not be thought of as a cure-all for all health related concerns. However, appropriate lifestyle, as described in this chapter, combined with consistent physical activity is a formula for success. As an individual, you have the opportunity to determine your own fate in relationship to the quality of life you will experience.

NOTES

[1]Gordon Edlin, *Health and Wellness,* 3rd ed. (Boston, MA: Jones and Bartlett Pub., 1988), p. 527.

[2]U.S. Public Health Service, Healthy People 2000: National Health Promotion and Disease Prevention Objectives, (Washington, D.C.: U.S. Government Printing Office, 1990).

[3] www.healthypeople.gov/

[4]*Sports Illustrated.* Sports Poll '86, Time, Inc. 1986.

[5]C.M. Brooks, "Adult Participation in Physical Activities Requiring Moderate to High levels of Energy Expenditure," The Physician and Sportsmedicine, XV (April, 1987), 118.

[6]K.E. Powell, "Physical Activity and the Incidence of Coronary Heart Disease," *Annual Review of Public Health,* VIII (1987), 253-287.

[7]J.F. Sallis, "Relation of Cardiovascular Fitness and Physical Activity to Cardiovascular Disease Risk Factors in Children and Adults," *American Journal of Epidemiology*, 127 (1988), 933-941.

[8]Edlin, p. 524.

[9]Aaron Wildavsky, "Doing Better and Feeling Worse: The Political Pathology of Health Policy," Daedalus, (Winter, 1976), 105-123.

[10]Surgeon General of the U.S., Healthy People, (Washington, DC.: U.S. Government Printing Office, 1979).

[11]*American College of Sport Medicine, Guidelines for Exercise Testing and Prescription,* 4th ed., (Philadelphia, PA: Lea and Febiger, 1991), p. 194.

[12]Werner K. Hoeger, Principles and Labs for Physical Fitness 2nd ed., (Englewood, CO: Morton Publishing, 1990), p. 43.

[13]ACSM, p. 196.

[14]William M. Kane, Healthy Living: An Active Approach to Wellness, (Indianapolis, IN: Bobbs-Merrill Publishing, 1985), p. 38.

[15]Kane, p. 67.

[16]E. Dawn McDonald, "Promoting Active Lifestyles Through Education," *Journal of Physical Education, Recreation, and Dance*, 64 (Jan., 1993), 37.

[17]Charles B. Corbin, Concepts of Physical Fitness, 7th ed., (Dubuque, IA: Wm. C. Brown Publishers, 1990), p. 237.

[18]Edlin, p. 528.

[19]Carl Gabbard, Lifelong Motor Development, (Dubuque, IA: Wm. C. Brown Publishers, 1992), p. 79.

[20]Everett L. Smith, "The Aging Process: Benefits of Physical Activity," Journal of Physical Education, Recreation, and Dance, 57 (Jan., 1986), p. 33.

Assessment of General Cardiovascular Fitness 2

"Cardiovascular fitness means the ability of the circulatory and respiratory systems to adjust to and recover from the effects of exercise or work."[1] How well the circulatory and respiratory systems adjust during exercise is directly proportional to the overall cardiovascular fitness of the individual. It is important for individuals to understand cardiovascular fitness levels in order to be successful in any type of exercise program.

The first essential step before embarking upon a successful aerobics program is to assess your general cardiovascular fitness level. This assessment is necessary in order to avoid starting an aerobics program in a haphazard way. In many cases, the individual starts training too hard in an aerobics program, which leaves one with a feeling of stress and thus without the desired outcome of optimum physical fitness. This type of unstructured approach often leads to the individual giving up jogging as a way of exercising.

It is important to note that if the individual is thirty years of age or older, a physical examination is recommended by a doctor before embarking upon an aerobics program. "The main objective of this examination is to spot heart, lung, and blood pressure problems that could make exercise potentially dangerous."[2] Individuals under thirty years of age can start exercising if they have been checked by a doctor in the past year and nothing was found wrong with them.

"Heart rate increases with oxygen consumption, and since the latter is considered to be the most valid measure of cardiorespiratory fitness, this relationship has been utilized in tests to predict oxygen consumption."[3] The heart rate of an individual can provide a great deal of information about adaptation to the stress of the exercise and is quick and easy to measure. This is the reason why so many evaluations about exercise are made by the measurement of the individual's heart rate. Factors that may influence an increase in the resting heart rate of an individual include temperature, humidity, previous activity, emotions, fatigue, infection, and time since eating or smoking. Thus,

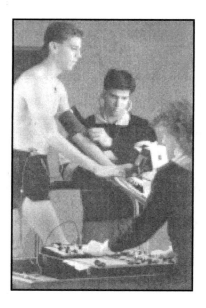

Figure 2.1
Treadmill Assessment of
Cardiovascular Fitness

resting heart rate is more variable than exercise and re-covery heart rates.[4]

The taking of pulse rates is best administered at either the radial or the carotid artery. The radial pulse is found in the hollow on the thumb side of the wrist about an inch from the base of the thumb. The carotid pulse is found just below the angle of the jaw on the neck. In both cases two fingers should be used to feel the pulse rather than a thumb, due to possible confusion of feeling one's own pulse rate transmitted through the thumb. It is important not to press too hard on the carotid artery as pressing too hard could cause an alteration in the heart beat and possi-bly in the breathing of the individual.[5] The individual counts the pulse rate for ten seconds, then multiplies that number times six to determine the pulse rate per minute.

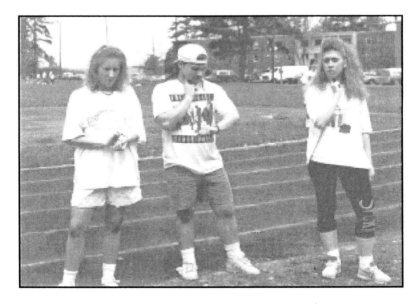

Figure 2.2
Taking the pulse rate

There are many tests available to assess cardiovascular fitness. To review all of them would not be appropriate for a beginning manual. The cardiovascular fitness test used most frequently for categorization purposes in an aerobics program is the 12-minute run–walk test.

RUN-WALK METHOD

The most commonly used method of assessing cardiovascular fitness is the run-walk method of testing. Of the run–walk test, Dr. Kenneth Cooper's 12-minute run–walk test is used most frequently because of its high validity factor of .94. (This means it measures, to a very high degree, what the test was designed to measure—cardiovascular fitness.)[6] For the purpose of this manual, the 12-minute run–walk test is used to assess cardiovascular fitness and determine the type of training program.

The objective of the 12-minute run–walk test is to cover the greatest distance possible in 12 minutes by running and/or walking if necessary. Dr. Kenneth Cooper developed tables to provide a breakdown of fitness from the results of the 12-minute run–walk test for both men and women.[7] In Chapter three of this text, there is a simplified table that can be used to assess cardiovascular fitness and to determine the beginning training level for the individual.

The 12-minute run–walk test is quite easy to administer. It is inexpensive to use and little equipment is needed. The only piece of equipment needed is a stopwatch for timing. If a track is not available, an open field can be measured and marked in order to administer the test properly. These markers should divide the course into quarters or eighths of a mile to make it easier to determine the distance covered in the test.

Something that needs to be stressed is the importance of pace judgment in taking the 12-minute run–walk test. By starting out too fast in the opening minutes of the test, a great amount of energy is expended that will hinder the performance of the individual for the remainder of the test. The objective of the test is to assess general cardiovascular fitness.

NOTES

[1]Barry L. Johnson, *Practical Measurements for Evaluation in Physical Education,* 3rd ed. (Minneapolis, Minnesota: Burgess Publishing Co., 1979), p. 142.

[2]Kenneth Cooper, *The New Aerobics* (New York: M. Evans and Co., 1970), p.22.

[3]Johnson, p. 143.

[4]George B. Dintiman, *Discovering Lifetime Fitness* (St. Paul, Minnesota: West Publishing, 1984), p. 4.

[5]Johnson, p. 158.

[6]T.L. Doolittle, "The Twelve-Minute Run-Walk: A Test of Cardiovascular Fitness of Adolescent Boys," *Research Quarterly,* XXXIX (October, 1968), 491-495.

[7]Kenneth Cooper, *The Aerobics Way* (New York: M. Evans and Company, 1977), p. 88.

KEEPING RECORDS

3

Figures 3.1 and 3.2 show the two areas of record keeping that need to be stressed in order to have a successful training regimen. The daily chart emphasizes the assessment of each individual workout so as to give the individual a clearer understanding of what particular objectives

---

Daily Training Chart

Date _____

Resting Pulse Rate _____

Post Exercise Pulse Rate:

    Immediately upon completion of exercise _____

    Five minutes after completion of exercise _____

Intensity of run (approximate time per mile) _____

Duration of run:

    Time _____

    Distance _____

Running Conditions:

    Weather _____

    Terrain _____

General Comments _____

_____

_____

_____

Figure 3.1

Monthly Training Chart
(In Miles)

Month _____

	Sunday	Monday	Tuesday	Wednesday	Thursday	Friday	Saturday	Weekly Total (Miles)
Week 1								
Week 2								
Week 3								
Week 4								
Week 5								

TOTAL MONTHLY MILES _____   TOTAL_____

Figure 3.2

were met for that particular workout. The monthly chart emphasizes the total picture of the long-range progress of the individual.

EXPLANATION OF THE BREAKDOWN OF DAILY RECORD KEEPING

Resting Pulse Rate

The heart rate at rest varies from individual to individual, so to determine a normal resting heart rate becomes very difficult. The average male heart rate is seventy-eight beats per minute, with women averaging five to ten beats faster than men. It is important to note also that taking the resting heart rate in the standing position as opposed to lying down can raise the heart rate ten to twelve beats per minute.[1] The importance of taking the resting heart rate is to monitor progress in the individual's condition. The better condition the individual attains, the lower the resting heart beat.

The key to taking the resting heart rate is standardization. The procedure must be consistent daily for the results to be valid. The best method to assure consistency is to take the pulse rate when you first wake up in the morning. This assures the same procedures daily and also builds in the necessity of lying down while taking the resting pulse rate for an accurate measurement.

Postexercise Pulse Rate

"The first two to three minutes after the end of the exercise, the heart rate decreases almost as rapidly as it increased."[2] This indicates the need for taking the pulse rate immediately after the completion of exercise to determine the workload of exercise. Sixty percent of the difference between the heart rate (220 heartbeats minus age) and the resting heart rate is considered the minimum for training benefit in the exercise.[3] Five minutes after the completion of the exercise, the pulse rate should be taken again and should be below 120 heart beats per minute. It should be noted that an unfit individual may not be able to train hard enough to get his/her heart rate above 120 heart beats per minute when first starting an aerobics program. The postexercise pulse rate is effective in measuring how strenuous the workout was, and how rapidly the body recovers from the fatigue of the exercise.

Intensity of Exercise

The intensity of the effort can be measured by two variables: the pace at which the individual covers a given distance, and the pulse rate of the individual. The pace at which the individual runs can be figured by taking the total time of the run and dividing it by the distance covered. (Example: 24 minutes divided by 3 miles = 8 minutes per mile pace). The pace factor is valid as long as variables such as weather conditions and terrain covered remain constant. Variations in such variables must be taken into account when comparing pace from one workout to another. Again, the pulse rate of the individual should be taken immediately upon completion of the exercise. The higher the pulse rate, the more intense the workout. It is important to note that individuals at low-fitness levels will benefit from a sustained effort of a heart rate at 120 beats per minute; whereas, an individual with a high fitness level would not benefit from sustained activity at 120 heart beats per minute.[4]

Duration of Run

The duration and intensity of the workout are closely interrelated in regard to aerobic effect. The two variables to be measured emphasizing the duration of the workout are the time it takes to complete the workout and the distance covered. An increase in either factor of pace or distance covered will show a positive aerobic effect. An example of this principle would be an individual at the low-fitness level. It would be wise to increase the duration of the workout for such an individual by walking intermittently so as to prolong the workout since the individual could not run very far in his/her condition of fitness at the beginning of a fitness program.

Running Conditions

Two primary variables that figure into the productivity of the workout are the weather and terrain. Extreme heat and cold will have an obvious effect on the workout of the individual. Also, factors such as wind, pollution, and humidity can have a definite effect on a workout. Different types of terrain can also have a definite effect on a workout. Hard surfaces such as roads are faster than soft surfaces such as grass. Hilly terrain will slow the pace down and increase the intensity of the workout proportionately. These variables should be recorded in the daily record-keeping process in order to add insight as to how the individual's training is coming along.

General Comments

This section is reserved for any additional insight that may be added that does not fit into any other appropriate category on the daily record keeping chart. This section should serve as an overall assessment of the workout completed. This accumulation of information can provide beneficial insight into the successful planning of future workouts on the basis of past successes and failures.

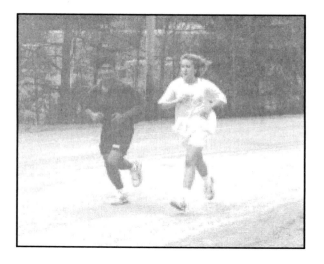

Figure 3.3
Hill Running

NOTES

[1]Hubert A. deVries, *Physiology of Exercise* (Dubuque, Iowa: W. C. Brown Co., 1980), p. 121.

[2]deVries, p. 122.

[3]deVries, p. 120.

[4]Michael L.Pollock, *Health and Fitness Through Physical Activity* (New York: John Wiley & Sons, 1978), p. 38.

Training Guide for a Successful Aerobics Program

4

Research indicates that three variables must be considered in designing any exercise program for developing cardiovascular fitness: frequency, intensity, and duration.[1] These three variables are not separate entities, but rather work together to form a positive correlation of a productive cardiovascular fitness program. A closer look at these three variables follows.

FREQUENCY

Naturally the optimum frequency for an aerobic program is daily participation. Research has indicated, however, that with as little as three training sessions a week, minimum aerobic gains can be attained.[2] Frequency alone, however, is not a valid method of determining aerobic benefit of an exercise program. Considerations of the intensity and duration of the individual training sessions must be considered along with frequency in order to measure the effect of the training.[3] Also, regularity of training must be taken into consideration when talking about frequency of training and the effect of training on cardiovascular fitness. If training is not a continuous and on-going process, the improvements gained diminish quite rapidly.[4] The higher the levels of frequency and regularity with correspondingly positive levels of intensity and duration, the higher the aerobic value of the training program. Individuals should strive toward a commitment of exercising as frequently as possible. At first, because of fatigue and initial soreness, it may be difficult to push yourself to the goal of daily training. With diligence and commitment this goal is attainable in a very short period of time.

INTENSITY

As previously mentioned in Unit 1, the minimum level for attaining a training effect is generally considered to be 60 percent of the difference between maximal and resting heart rate. "For unfit individuals and middle-aged and older persons, the minimal training threshold may be as low as 100 to 120 beats per minute."[5] The improvement of aerobic capacity is directly proportional to the intensity level of training. It is important that individuals be aware of their fitness level so that they can wisely determine an intensity level of training that can increase their aerobic capacity without over-exertion and frustration. In determining the intensity level of training, it is better to underestimate one's capabilities and start out too easy rather than overestimate one's capabilities and over-extend the body. A slower, more gradual approach in increasing the intensity level of training is best for the individual physiologically and psychologically.

DURATION

The duration of training is closely related to the intensity level of training. Research has indicated that improvement in aerobic capacity has been shown with moderate to high level intensity training lasting only five to ten minutes daily.[6] For the average adult in our society, a minimum of ten to fifteen minutes of exercise is required to improve aerobic capacity.[7] The duration of the training is in direct proportion to the intensity level. As the intensity level increases, the length of the training period decreases to attain the same aerobic effect and vice versa. The more practical method to use in starting an aerobics program is to lower the intensity level of training and to increase the duration of training. For most individuals this would mean starting with a program that includes periods of walking for recuperation so as to extend the duration of the exercise for maximum benefit.

In setting up a training program, it is important to realize that no one training program will fit everyone's needs. It is important to realize that we are all individuals, and needs differ according to lifestyle, fitness levels and many other variables. This brings us to the important variable of flexibility. Individuals must be flexible in their training schedule so that when circumstances arise that prohibit following the schedule, alterations can be made to derive similar benefits. An example of this might be that because of fatigue, an individual may take a training day off or train easily for the day. "Fatigue is a sign that your body is not ready to be stressed."[8] The body must be allowed to recover from this feeling of fatigue to eliminate the risk of potential injury.

Another important principle to follow for a successful aerobics program is that of gradualism. An aerobics program should be one that concentrates on steady and sensible improvement of training patterns. "Consider that you are in training to develop a habit of permanent moderate exercise."[9] The permanent aspect of training is essential to derive positive benefits from your program. The most efficient methods to assure permanency in a training program is the gradual method involving slow but steady progress toward increasing the intensity and duration of training. This can be accomplished by starting slowly, and "training, not straining."[10]

"The main objective of an aerobic exercise program is to increase the maximum amount of oxygen that the body can process within a given time."[11] Dr. Kenneth Cooper advocates that a number of activities such as swimming, cycling, rowing, and jogging can be used to produce these desired effects. The most efficient method of increasing the duration of jogging is to have short pauses of walking intermittently for recovery purposes.[12] Many individuals starting an aerobics program are only able to jog for very short periods of time. Short periods of walking mixed with jogging will enable an individual to increase the duration of the training period.

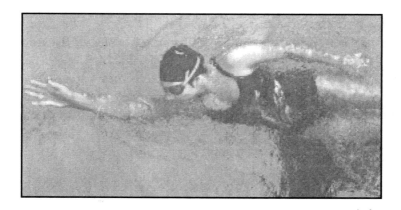

Figure 4.1
Swimming

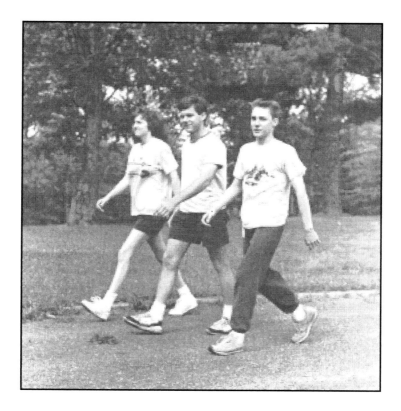

Figure 4.2
Walking

Another principle important to adhere to in starting an aerobics program is to prepare for a period of gradual adjustment to vigorous exercise. "As should be the case for any strenuous activity, a period of several weeks of easy running should precede any attempts of a vigorous training schedule of any kind."[13]

A pretraining period is valuable for injury prevention and mental adjustment to regular training. The first few weeks are needed to make adjustments to a new form of exercising. This pretraining period is excellent for breaking into a regular training schedule while avoiding the risk of injury. A gradual approach leads to successful transition of mental adjustment necessary for regularity in the individual's training program.

After completing the initial assessment of general cardiovascular endurance by taking the 12-minute run–walk test, attention can now be directed toward setting up a training schedule. Most individuals will experience improvement in the first couple of months of training, so intermediate and overall assessment can be scheduled appropriately, although the training should be set up to be flexible enough to be followed in any time span.

To determine what training level to start with, the individual can consult the following breakdown from the 12-minute run–walk test:

Distance covered in miles	Level
−1.0	1
1.0 −1.25	2
1.25–1.50	3
1.50–1.75	4
1.75 and up	5

In all levels the 12-minute test can be retaken at any time to assess progress of the training program. If the individual progresses into a higher category, the training schedule can be adjusted accordingly. It is important to note that an individual should not become discouraged if he does not progress to a higher level within the first couple of months of training. An individual that is sincere and diligent about training will experience positive results that often cannot be measured on a chart.

LEVEL ONE

If you covered less than one mile in twelve minutes, you are classified as being in very poor physical condition. It is important to realize you are in very poor condition, so that you understand that it is going to be a long and gradual process to attain optimum physical fitness. An individual in this condition should start by doing a lot of walking and very little jogging. As the individual progresses into better condition, the amount of walking will decrease, and the amount of jogging will increase. The important variable is the duration of the exercise. At this level, twenty minutes a day will produce positive results. As the condition of the individual improves, the greater the distance he will cover in that twenty-minute period.[14]

The intensity level of work should be very light at first. The individual should feel for the first couple of weeks that he is not working hard enough, so as to give the body a chance to adjust and get over the initial soreness and fatigue. Any time the individual is running and feels that he is winded to the point he could not talk to the individual next to him, he should walk for a while to recover. It is important to note that if the individual is obese, this will slow down the progress of an aerobics program. "Since energy output relates directly to body weight, heavier people burn more calories (and therefore use more oxygen in the process) for a given type of exertion than thin people."[15] Excess weight will obviously cause more work on the cardiovascular system, thus using more energy to do less work. It is imperative that obese individuals strive to lose weight along with working out regularly.

LEVEL TWO

Individuals fitting into this classification are very similar to Plan A in that they are in poor physical condition and have a long gradual road ahead of them to obtain optimum physical fitness. The individual at this level will probably be able to start alternating jogging and walking about equally depending upon whether he is closer to 1.0 mile in twelve minutes or 1.25 miles in twelve minutes. Again, a duration of twenty minutes is sufficient to produce positive desired benefits. More than twenty minutes per workout runs the danger of over-work and fatigue of the body. As the individual attains better physical condition, he will be able to do more jogging in the workout, thus covering more distance in each workout.

The intensity level again should start very lightly for the period of adjustment of the body to exercise, and very gradually increase without putting undue strain upon the body. The key to the intensity level is consistency in training. If an individual works too hard forcing days of recovery from over-exertion, the training will not be as beneficial as the slower, more gradual build-up approach. The more gradual approach is also much better for the individual's psychological outlook on the program.

LEVEL THREE

An individual starting in this classification is considered to be in fair cardiovascular condition. This classification by no means states that the individual is ready to exercise hard for extended periods of time. An individual at this level of fitness probably can handle about twice as much jogging as walking during a workout. The individual in this category can exercise for twenty-five minutes during a workout at a moderate level of intensity without putting undue stress upon the body. The key again lies in the fact that the individual needs to listen to the body and ease off the pace when his body tells him that he is going too fast.

This is the level into which most people fit. Many individuals make the mistake of wanting to quickly increase the intensity and duration of the workouts once they get over the initial soreness and fatigue of starting the program. This leads to injuries, a negative attitude toward jogging, and possible discontinuance of the program. A slower and more gradual approach is more sensible and easier to maintain over a long period of time.

LEVEL FOUR

An individual fitting into this category is considered to be in good to excellent (depending on age and sex) cardiovascular condition. Individuals fitting into this category generally have either been running prior to starting an aerobics program, or have been participating regularly in some type of physically demanding exercise program. An individual in this category is generally ready to exercise for about thirty minutes daily without undue fatigue or strain to the body. The intensity level should again be moderate. Although it is not uncommon for individuals at this level to be able to jog for thirty minutes without stopping, it may be wise to occasionally walk intermittently throughout the workout. A common mistake for individuals in this classification is the desire to attain the excellent level of cardiovascular fitness too hurriedly. Again, the slower more gradual approach is the sensible approach to attaining this optimum level.

LEVEL FIVE

An individual attaining this classification is beyond the beginning stage of jogging as a form of aerobic exercise. Some individuals are blessed with a superior cardiovascular system but do not understand the basic principles of successfully setting up a training program. An individual in this classification can reasonably handle a minimum of thirty minutes of exercise daily. The intensity level should range from moderately light to moderately hard. Intensity and duration of the workout combine to determine the extent the individual should work. An increase of either the intensity or duration beyond the normal working capacity is considered to be a "hard day" workout, which should be followed by an "easy day" workout of lessening either the intensity or duration is necessary. This type of "hard day" — "easy day" rotation is considered valid in maximizing training, while still allowing the body to recover.

It is extremely important at all five levels to stay in tune with what your body is telling you regarding the intensity of the training session. Under-training is more sensible and healthful than over-extending one's body limits and risking possible injury in addition to mental anguish which frequently accompanies over-training. Again, the key concept to remember is gradualism regarding training patterns.

NOTES

[1]I. E. Faria, I"Cardiovascular Response to Exercise as Influenced by Training of Various Intensities," *Research Quarterly,* XLI (March, 1970), 44; Donald K. Mathews, *The Physiological Basis of Physical Education and Athletics,* 2nd ed. (Philadelphia: W.B. Saunders Co., 1976), p.52.

[2]Charles Corbin, *Concepts in Physical Education,* 7th ed. (Dubuque, Iowa: Brown Co., 1990), p. 46.

[3]Michael Pollock, *Health and Fitness Through Physical Activity* (New York: John Wiley & Sons, 1978), p. 40.

[4]Werner W. Hoeger, *Lifetime Physical Fitness and Wellness,* 3rd ed., (Englewood, CO: Morton Publishing Co., 1992).

[5]Pollock, p. 38.

[6]Pollock, p. 38.

[7]Corbin, p. 47.

[8]Jack Daniels, *Conditioning for Distance Running* (New York: John Wiley & Sons, 1978), p. 58.

[9]William J. Bowerman, *Jogging* (New York: Carter, 1967), p. 52.

[10]Bowerman, p. 31.

[11]Kenneth H. Cooper, *The New Aerobics* (New York: M. Evans & Co., 1970), p. 16.

[12]Ernst Van Aaken, *The Van Aaken Method* (Mt. View, Ca.: World Publications, Inc., 1976), p. 60.

[13]Daniels, p. 59.

[14]Pollock, p. 38.

[15]Robert Buxbaum, *Sports for Life* (Boston: Beacon Press, 1979), p. 20.

TRAINING SESSION PREPARATION PHASE   **5**

The preparatory phase before the actual start of the training session is more commonly referred to as the "warm-up." The warm-up generally consists of two variables, easy jogging and flexibility-type stretching exercises. It is important to emphasize that the warm-up is done at a low intensity level. The importance of a good warm-up period centers around the need to gradually prepare the body for the training session. "Research has shown that blood flow to critical areas (such as the heart) does not increase immediately."[1]

> The warmup allows the heart to increase its rate per minute and volume per beat so that adequate amounts of oxygenated blood reach the working muscles. It allows muscle and body temperature to rise slightly, which provide for an optimal metabolic and physiological environment. The warmup also allows time for fat to be released from its storage sites into the blood so that the working muscles can utilize it.[2]

The essential attributes of a good warm-up center around injury prevention and preparation of the body for physical exertion. The amount of time needed for a proper warmup will vary depending on the individual's needs, but approximately fifteen minutes used wisely will usually be sufficient. An example of an efficient method of warming up is approximately five minutes of easy jogging, another seven to ten minutes of flexibility exercises, then a few more minutes of easy jogging. Again, it is important to keep the intensity level low on the warmup and the duration of the easy jogging should be proportional to the fitness condition level of the individual. The warm-up is done to prepare the individual for the training session, not for training benefit or to fatigue the individual.

The aspect of flexibility of the individual is a widely misunderstood variable. "Flexibility can be most simply defined as the range of possible movement in a joint or series of joints."[3] Size of the individual has little or no effect on the flexibility of the individual. For example, there is no relationship between leg length or trunk length of the individual and the scores made on flexibility tests.[4] Some factors that do affect flexibility are age, sex, activity, and temperature.[5] A child's flexibility increases until adolescence; then the level of flexibility decreases progressively with age. So, as the individual gets older, greater emphasis must be placed on appropriate exercises to increase flexibility. Women are more flexible than men due to anatomical differences in the joints and to the type of physical activities the two sexes tend to choose. Active individuals tend to be more flexible than inactive individuals. Muscles that are not used regularly are maintained in a shortened position and lose mobility. A raised temperature of the muscles will increase the degree of flexibility and proportionally the lowered temperature will decrease the degree of flexibility.

To increase flexibility, the two types of stretching exercises most commonly used are ballistic and static stretching. The ballistic stretch involves a bouncing or jerking motion to gain momentum in the body part in order to stretch farther.[6] The static stretch is a slow sustained stretching exercise that places a muscle in a lengthened position and holds the position for a few seconds.[7] Both the ballistic and static stretch use the overload principle of stretching the muscle beyond its normal length. Both methods are effective in increasing flexibility if used regularly and properly. It is important to note that the overdevelopment of one muscle group while neglecting the opposing muscle group results in an imbalance that restricts flexibility.[8] The balance of a good stretching system is important which leads the writer to further investigation of the positive and negative attributes of ballistic and static stretching.

BALLISTIC STRETCH

The ballistic stretch works on the principle of utilizing momentum to provide the overloading effect to the joints necessary to increase flexibility. The opposing muscle groups usually produce the movement necessary for a ballistic stretch, so there is a balance of both the muscle group and its opposing muscle group being worked in the ballistic type of stretch. Because large muscle groups are easily worked into a ballistic stretch, it is generally more effective on trunk and leg flexibility. The major problem most individuals encounter with ballistic stretching is that they tend to overstretch, which tends to cause injury especially in the presence of an old injury where scar tissue is present.

STATIC STRETCH

The static stretch involves the principle of working against a force greater than that of opposing muscle groups in order to stretch the desired muscles. This force usually is either a partner or an outside force such as a wall, tree, etc., in which the individual exerts force. This type of stretch places individuals in situations where they are less likely to overstretch possibly causing soreness or injury. Static stretching can also be used to help shin splints as well as relieve soreness to muscles in the calf and quadriceps.[9] The primary limitation with the static stretch is its failure to work the opposing muscle groups. This creates the necessity to supplement static stretching with ballistic stretching and to make sure that static stretching is used in the opposing muscle groups. The static stretch is also less effective in relationship to trunk and leg flexibility.

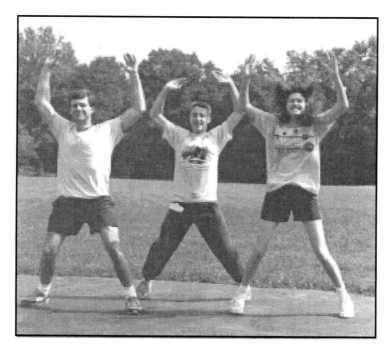

Figure 5.1
Ballistic stretching

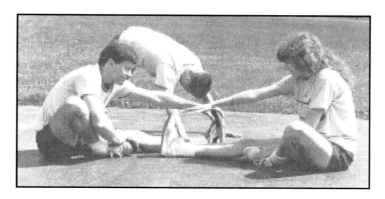

Figure 5.2
Static stretching

The following is a list of guidelines for performing flexibility exercises using both ballistic and static stretching:[10]

1. Avoid ballistic exercises of previously injured muscles.
2. When ballistic stretching is used, bounces should be easy and gentle movements to avoid over-stretching.
3. Static stretching should be repeated several times daily.
4. Static stretching should be held from six to twelve seconds.
5. To increase flexibility, the muscle must be stretched beyond normal length.

The length of the warm-up will center around the weather conditions and flexibility of the individual. The cooler the weather condition, the longer the warm-up period will need to be. Flexibility is important for injury prevention and to prepare the body to comfortably start the training session. Individuals with poor levels of flexibility should spend more time concentrated in this area for needed improvements.

The jogging phase of the warmup should be done prior to the flexibility exercises and again upon the completion of the flexibility stretching. The easy jogging prior to the stretching exercises is excellent because it increases the temperature of the body and its muscles. The easy jogging following the completion of the stretching exercises is important in order to prepare the body for the gradual transition into the training session. For individuals in better condition, a few seventy to eighty-yard wind sprints might be added before starting the training session. A wind sprint is a run of approximately seventy to eighty yards where the individual gradually increases his speed to approximately 75 percent of top speed for the latter portion of the distance. Wind sprints should be done in a way that avoids a jerking start that provides an initial burst of speed similar to that of a sprinter. Instead, an even acceleration should take place so that the individual at the latter stages of the wind sprint attains the desired optimum speed.

NOTES

[1]Grath A. Fisher, *The Complete Book of Physical Fitness* (Provo, Utah: Brigham Young University Press, 1979), p. 10.

[2]Jack Daniels, *Conditioning for Distance Running* (New York: John Wiley & Sons, 1978), pp. 58-59.

[3]Hubert A. deVries, *Physiology of Exercise* (Dubuque, Iowa: Wm. C. Brown Co., 1980), p. 462.

[4]M. L. Harris, "A Factor Analysis of Flexibility," *Research Quarterly,* XL (March, 1969), 62.

[5]deVries, p. 368.

[6]Charles Corbin, *Concepts in Physical Education* 7th ed., (Dubuque, Iowa: W.C. Brown Co., 1990), p. 73.

[7]Corbin, p. 74.

[8]W. F. Updyke, *Principles of Modern Physical Education, Health and Recreation* (New York: Holt, Rinehart, and Winston Inc., 1970), p. 47.

[9]Hubert A. deVries, "Prevention of Muscular Distress After Exercise," *Research Quarterly,* XXXII (May, 1961), 177.

[10]Corbin, p. 78.

TRAINING SESSION RECOVERY PHASE

6

The recovery phase of the training session is commonly referred to as the "cooling down" period following the workout. The cooling down period is an important part of the training session for the safety and well-being of the individual. During moderate exercise, the "muscle pumping" action can account for as much as 40 percent of the blood pumping in the body. "During cardiovascular work, the muscles squeeze the veins rhythmically, helping the blood return to the heart."[1] If an individual were to stop suddenly and proceed with no physical activity, this would cause the heart to do all the pumping alone. This can lead to a sudden decreased volume of blood to the brain, which on occasion has caused joggers to pass out while standing waiting for a signal light to turn green.

Another problem that must be dealt with during the cooling down period is the working out of lactic acid in the muscles. Lactic acid forms in the muscles during the workout, resulting in blood of an acidic nature.[2] It is important to replenish this acidic blood in the muscles with blood of a lower acidic balance. The most efficient way of doing this is by stimulating the circulation of the blood by increasing oxygen to this transport system without causing an oxygen debt (lack of oxygen to vital organs). The easiest method of accomplishing this is to jog easily for a few minutes upon the completion of the training session.

If lactic acid is not worked out of the muscles, it will pool in the muscles causing soreness and stiffness.

Flexibility stretching is also important at the completion of the training session. A higher temperature of muscles is required in order to stretch the muscle to improve flexibility. Following the training session is an ideal time to work on increased flexibility because of the definite rise in muscle temperature. Also, stretching exercises are excellent for prevention of sore muscles and joints. Massaging the muscles has limited benefits because of the lack of circulatory effect of the acidic blood away from the muscles.[3] Jogging is more efficient because it has the benefit of increasing supplies of oxygen for circulatory purposes. Stretching exercises will also create greater circulatory benefits than massaging.

Unfortunately, many joggers neglect to properly cool down or fail to see the value of a proper cooling down period. Neglecting to cool down properly can result in injury and illness. An individual that neglects the cooling down period may suffer soreness and stiffness. Also, by neglecting to follow proper cooling down techniques, the individual is missing an opportune time to increase flexibility and diminish the chance of future injuries.

NOTES

[1]Grath A. Fisher, *The Complete Book of Physical Fitness* (Provo, Utah: Brigham Young University Press, 1979), p. 10.

[2]Arthur Lydiard, *Running the Lydiard Way* (Mt. View, Ca.: World Publications, Inc., 1978), p. 87.

[3]Lydiard, p. 88.

NUTRITION
AS RELATED TO AEROBICS

7

"There is no scientific evidence at the present time to indicate that athletic performance can be improved by modifying a basically sound diet."[1] The key here is "sound diet." If the individual is on a sound diet, special emphasis on a particular area of an individual's diet will generally have only a psychological effect, yet in reality cause no alterations necessary to positively enhance physical performance levels.

Caloric intake is important for a well-balanced diet. There are many factors that determine the number of calories needed per day such as age, sex, size, glandular function, emotional state, climate, exercise intensity level, etc. The exercise intensity level is very important in relationship to diet because the individual must consume enough calories daily to meet the energy demands of the training schedule. A moderately active college-age woman needs about 2,000 calories per day, while a moderately active man of that age needs about 2,800 calories per day. A female athlete in training may burn from 2,600 calories to 3,500 calories daily; whereas a male athlete in training may burn from 3,500 calories to 5,500 calories daily. An individual consuming less calories than he/she is using up during training will start burning body tissues to make up the deficit, causing "staleness" and increasing the likelihood of injury.[2]

Important to nutrition in relationship to exercise is that of the proportion of the different kinds of nutrients necessary for the body to adjust properly to the demands of exercise. There are six general classes of nutrients necessary for the body to function properly: carbohydrates, fats, proteins, vitamins, minerals, and water. "Carbohydrates, fats and proteins are often spoken of as the fuel or energy nutrients, since they are the only substances that the body can use to supply energy for work and heat."[3] A further examination of these three nutrients in relationship to exercising is in order.

CARBOHYDRATES

Carbohydrates are the most abundant nutrient found in food. Carbohydrates are not only the most economical source of energy, but also the major source of energy when it comes to exercising.[4] Carbohydrates provide most of the energy during exercising of moderate to heavy intensity levels and for prolonged periods of time requiring about 75 percent maximum working capacity.[5] Some of the more common sources of carbohydrates are grain products, fruits, nuts, vegetables, dried fruits, maple syrups and starchy food products.

FATS

Fats are the most concentrated source of energy available. Fats contain approximately twice as many calories as do carbohydrates, but do not produce twice the energy that carbohydrates do. Most individuals consume approximately 40 percent of their calories in fats. For health and weight control reasons, an individual would be wiser to consume only 25 percent of his/her calories through fats.[6] Some common examples of fats are butter, margarine, vegetable oils, lard, and suet. Considering the high caloric value of fats, it becomes obvious that fats are not a source that an individual desires to over-indulge in to attain extra energy sources for training purposes.

PROTEIN

Protein provides the amino acids that are essential to the building and growth of new tissues and provides an alternate source of energy. "If the dietary amount of fat and carbohydrate is sufficient, then just a small amount of high-quality protein is needed for an adult—approximately 8 to 9 percent of the total daily calories."[7] Supplements to protein needs are generally not needed for active individuals, because with a well-balanced diet, as caloric intake increases more protein is consumed. "Total deprivation of protein with adequate energy intake for two weeks has not been shown to alter performance of fixed work tasks in a laboratory nor to reduce muscular strength."[8] Good protein sources are generally considered to be eggs, milk, meat, fish, and poultry. Increased levels of protein are recommended for infants, children, pregnant or lactating women.

Concerning the timing of the consumption of these nutrients; it is widely accepted that the caloric intake be evenly spread out over the course of a day. Research has indicated that more frequent intake of smaller amounts of food may be desirable for individuals participating in vigorous physical activities. "Omission of breakfast does lead to poorer work performance, and blood sugar falls to undesirably low levels with continued deprivation of food."[9]

Approximately one-fourth of the day's calories should be consumed at breakfast. Individuals who do not eat breakfast generally over-eat in other meals to make up the needed calories for daily activity use, which goes against the principle of evenly spreading calorie consumption during the day for optimum exercise benefit and weight control. In regard to eating before a training session, it takes approximately three to four hours to digest a normal meal.[10] The digestion of food takes place in proportion to the amount and type of foods ingested. Before a workout, caution should be taken to avoid eating foods that you know are hard for your body system to digest.

Many individuals begin an aerobics program for the primary purpose of losing weight. There are generally two classifications for individuals, needing to lose weight or being overweight or obese. "Overweight means being above average weight, while being obese means having deposits of excessive body fat."[11] Overweight and obesity may be caused by any number of reasons ranging from poor eating habits, overeating and lack of exercise to glandular and other conditions of the body that do not reflect negative lifestyles. Individuals that are overweight or obese due to reasons other than overeating and/or lack of exercise should obtain medical advice before starting any reducing program. In any weight-reducing program, the weight should be taken off gradually with care taken to ensure that all essential nutrients are included in adequate amounts in the reducing program.

To lose weight, an individual must increase calorie expenditure through activity or reduce intake of calories through diet. A combination of these two methods is most effective over the long run because this method does not alter normal living patterns. Most individuals who attempt fad or crash diets may see significant early results, but because of the drastic change of lifestyle, are not able to stick with the diet and put the weight lost back on as quickly as they lost it. The combined reduction of just five hundred calories a day through activity expenditure and diet would mean the loss of a pound a week, which most individuals can handle for extended periods of time. There are circumstances in which obese individuals may actually gain weight when first starting an aerobics program. Because they are low in strength and muscular develop-ment, body fat is lost but is replaced by muscle tissue, which weighs more than fat. Although the individual has not lost weight, the change of body composition to more fat-free weight should accomplish a trimmer appearance.[12]

Body composition is not only important from a health standpoint, but the lower the percentage of body fat in the individual, the more efficiently the cardiovascular system operates. This variable becomes important with age. The percentage of body fat of an individual generally increases steadily after the age of twenty because of more sedentary living habits. Exercise has been shown to be effective in off-setting and/or delaying this trend.[13] Many individuals in our society are also concerned about spot reducing in areas such as hips, midsection, etc. Spot reducing may be effective but probably no more than general "nonspot" ex-ercise of equal intensity and duration.[14] Most positive re-sults can be attributed to the development of better muscle tone involved in all supporting areas, not the specific area alone.

NOTES

[1]Hubert A. deVries, *Physiology of Exercise* (Dubuque, Iowa: Brown Co., 1980), p. 522.

[2]A. Grath Fisher, *Scientific Basis of Athletic Conditioning* (Philadelphia: Lea and Febiger, 1990), p. 205.

[3]L. Jean Bogert, L*Nutrition and Physical Fitness,* 9th ed. (Philadelphia: W. B. Saunders Co., 1973), p. 8.

[4]Lilnda Garrison, *Fitness and Figure Control,* 2nd ed. (Palo Alto, Ca.: Mayfield Publishing Co., 1981), p. 11.

[5]D. W. Edington, *The Biology of Physical Activity* (Boston: Houghton Mifflin Co., 1976), p. 255.

[6]Melvin H. Williams, *Lifetime Fitness and Wellness* (Dubuque, Iowa: Wm. C. Brown, 1990), p. 217.

[7]Marie Krause, *Food Nutrition and Diet Therapy* (Philadelphia: W. B. Saunders, 1979), p. 82.

[8]Bogert, p. 489.

[9]Bogert, p. 490.

[10]Charles Corbin, *Concepts in Physical Education* 7th ed., (Dubuque, Iowa: W.C. Brown Co., 1990), p. 226.

[11]Harold B. Falls, *Foundations of Conditioning* (New York: Academic Press, 1970), p. 153.

[12]Lon H. Seiger, *Walking for Fitness* (Dubuque, Iowa: Wm. C. Brown, 1990), p. 91.

[13]Joan Luckman, *Your Health* (Englewood Cliffs, New Jersey: Prentice Hall, 1990), p. 80.

[14]M. L. Carns, "Segmental Volume Reduction by Localized versus Generalized Exercise," *Human Biology,* XXXII (1960), 370-376.

Physiological Basis for Cardiovascular Fitness 8

The physiological effects of training on an individual are many and varied. The maintenance of good cardiovascular fitness is a complex issue because it requires proper fitness of so many different systems and their functions in the body. An aerobics program would have an obvious positive effect upon the efficiency of the respiratory (lungs) and cardiovascular (heart and blood vessels) systems, but other effects such as gains in muscular strength and endurance would be developed in such areas as the legs and trunk of the individual.[1] To discuss all the physiological components that relate to cardiovascular fitness would be out of context for a beginning manual. This unit will primarily center around the functions of the heart and oxygen transport systems.

Effects of Physical Training Upon the Heart and Circulatory System

Changes to the heart and circulatory system induced by training include the following:

Increased—Size of heart, efficiency and strength, stroke volume, hemoglobin, blood volume, ability to handle stress, and cardiac output.

Decreased—Resting heart rate, strokes per minute, blood pressure (if individual is considered

to be hypertensive), incidence of heart disease, cholesterol, and triglycerides.

HEART SIZE

The heart is a muscle, so with training it will grow in
size. "By training a muscle, including the heart, gradually
and carefully over a period of time, its efficiency and
strength can be increased many times over."[2] This increase
in strength and efficiency of the heart is important because
of the increased stroke volume capabilities of the individual with fewer strokes per minute. Increased stroke volume permits more blood and oxygen to reach the muscles
necessary for successful training. Heredity is important in
determination of size of heart and other essential aerobic
capacities; but in tests of identical twins with similar physical characteristics, endurance training can account for as
much as a 20 percent difference in aerobic capacity.[3] This
indicates that with training, any individual can increase
the strength and efficiency of his/her heart in relationship
to endurance training. At the present time, research has
found no evidence that regular progressive exercise is bad
for the normal heart, thus contradicting the so-called "athlete's heart" myth that strenuous work harms the heart.[4]

HEART RATE

A common trait experienced by individuals involved
in endurance training is the lowering of their pulse rates. A
slower heart rate is accompanied by a greater stroke
volume, thus indicating a stronger and more efficient
heart. In using the resting heart rate as a criterion for fitness, one must give consideration to the wide variability of

range within the general population.[5] Thus, it becomes important to compare progress in the area of resting pulse rate with the individual himself, and not with statistics of the general population because of the wide range of variability. Two variables need to be taken into consideration in regard to decrease of resting heart rate: one is the fact that for many individuals, it will require training for a long period of time to have a profound effect on the resting heart rate; one other variable is that the magnitude of the decrease produced by training is less when the level of fitness is greater.[6]

STROKE VOLUME

The stroke volume is the amount of blood pumped out of the heart per beat. The stroke volume for distance runners has been reported to be nearly double that of the normal population.[7] The positive effect of increased stroke volume of the heart is the increase of blood and oxygen to the muscles, enabling the muscles to work for longer periods of time more efficiently. Larger stroke volume is a result of an increased ventricular cavity, thus allowing more blood to fill the ventricle during diastole (recovery portion of the heart beat).[8] This enables more blood being pumped each stroke, thus enabling fewer strokes per minute to do the work. Greater stroke volume enables the individual to achieve greater oxygen-carbon dioxide exchange, resulting in more available oxygen taken from the air and also a lower rate of lactic acid formation in the individual.[9]

BLOOD VOLUME AND HEMOGLOBIN

Both the total blood volume and hemoglobin increase with training.[10] The significance of this increase is the positive correlation between maximum oxygen uptake with the increase in blood volume and hemoglobin levels. The blood volume transport system in the hemoglobin transports the oxygen through the blood to the muscles. Training at moderate levels of intensity will increase the blood volume and hemoglobin levels from 20 to 25 percent.[11]

Some benefits to the heart system derived from continuous physical training include the following:

1. Reduction of blood pressure of individuals that are considered hypertensive (individuals with normal blood pressure generally show little or no effect with training).[12]

2. Lower incidence of heart disease.[13]

3. Effective prescription for those who have suffered heart attacks.[14]

4. Heart rate returns to normal faster after emotional stress and the individual is better equipped to handle stress.[15]

CHANGES IN CHOLESTEROL AND TRIGLYCERIDE LEVELS

"Regular exercise programs cause decreases in both blood cholesterol and triglyceride levels."[16] The effects of excessive amounts of cholesterol in the bloodstream are well known; it clogs the arteries and increases the likelihood of stroke and heart disease. This change is more pronounced in individuals with very high levels prior to starting an exercise program. Exercise is the most efficient method to ensure there will not be a build up of cholesterol and triglycerides, thus slowing down the flow of blood in the arteries.

EFFECTS OF PHYSICAL TRAINING UPON THE RESPIRATORY SYSTEM

Changes induced to the respiratory system by training include the following:

Increased — Lung capacity, breathing capacity, oxygen to skeletal muscles, maximum oxygen uptake, diffusion capacity, myoglobin, oxidation of carbohydrates and fats.

Decreased — Oxygen to respiratory muscles and lactic acid accumulation.

PULMONARY VENTILATION

Training causes an increase in both the total lung volume and minimum breathing capacity. Pulmonary functions are considered secondary to the capacity of the heart and circulation, and cellular functions. Arterial blood leaing the heart is approximately 97 percent saturated with oxygen, unless the individual is training at higher altitudes (causing less air available to breathe) or the individual has a respiratory ailment preventing normal breathing.[17] Pulmonary factors very seldom limit endurance performance because the heart and its circulatory process determine maximum oxygen uptake.

VENTILATORY EFFICIENCY

Training causes an increased ventilatory efficiency. The amount of air ventilated for trained individuals is lower, thus being a more efficient respiratory system. This is accomplished by less oxygen going to respiratory muscles and more oxygen going to the working skeletal muscles.[18] Increases in efficiency of the working skeletal muscles are essential for endurance capabilities for prolonged periods of time. This is accomplished by providing more oxygen into the circulatory process for maximum operating efficiency of the skeletal muscles.

MAXIMAL OXYGEN UPTAKE

"Maximal oxygen uptake is the greatest amount of oxygen a person can take in during exercise and so reflects his ability to transport oxygen to his tissues."[19] Aerobic training increases the muscle mass in the chest cavity, thus increasing the oxygen consumption capabilities of the individual. Weight of the individual must be taken into consideration when considering maximal oxygen uptake. Frequently a heavier individual will have a larger muscle mass in the chest cavity enabling more oxygen consumption, yet be less efficient in maximal oxygen uptake because of increased demands on the respiratory system to provide the necessary fuel to move larger masses. Increased oxygen consumption enables the more complete breakdown of glycogen (carbohydrates) in the muscle tissues. The more complete the glycogen breakdown, the less the accumulation of lactic acid in the working muscle tissue, thus a more efficient working body system. It is important to note that the elimination of lactic acid is impossible, but through continuous training, lactic acid accumulation takes longer to set in and can be worked out much more easily in the "warmdown" session at the completion of the workout.

DIFFUSION CAPACITY

In any aerobic activity, it is essential that the oxygen coming into the body be efficiently transmitted from the membrane system through diffusion to the circulatory system. Through training, the diffusion capacity of the individual is increased by more efficient cellular systems and larger lung volume. Utilization of the oxygenated blood being transported throughout the body by red blood cells is done more efficiently in trained individuals. Metabolism of carbon dioxide and lactic acid, so important in participation in endurance activities, is done more efficiently in trained individuals.[20] Increased lung volume enables the body to efficiently handle greater volumes of oxygen necessary for endurance activities.

Some benefits to the respiratory system derived from continuous physical training include the following:

1. Increase of myoglobin content—Myoglobin is an oxygen-binding pigment similar to hemoglobin that acts as a store for oxygen.[21]

2. Increased oxidation of carbohydrates—This increases the capacity of the muscle to generate energy aerobically. As mentioned in Unit 6, carbohydrates are the primary source of energy for aerobic activities.

3. Increased oxidation of fat—Similar to carbohydrates, the oxidation process of fats is more effi-

cient, allowing better utilization of this major energy source.

EFFECTS OF PHYSICAL TRAINING UPON THE BODY

Changes induced to the overall body by training include the following:

Increased — Lean body weight (slight or no change) and heat acclimatization.

Decreased — Total body fat and total body weight.

CHANGES IN BODY COMPOSITION

The following changes in body composition frequently occur with moderate levels of exercising:

1. A decrease in total body fat,
2. No change or slight increase in lean body weight,
3. A small decrease in total body weight.[22]

These changes, particularly that of loss of weight, are more pronounced for men and women that are obese as opposed to individuals already "lean." As mentioned in Unit 6, loss of body fat is dependent upon the balance between caloric intake and caloric expenditure through exercise.

HEAT ACCLIMATIZATION

Heat acclimatization is increased by training, due to the body's ability to adapt to the physiological adjustments necessary to adapt to the stress of high temperatures. This is true even if the training is not being carried out in hot environments. "Heat acclimatization promoted by physical training apparently is stimulated by the large amounts of heat produced during the training sessions."[23] This increase in heat causes a rise in skin and body temperature comparable to that which would be encountered while training in hot environments.

NOTES

[1]Michael Pollock, *Health and Fitness Through Physical Activity* (New York: John Wiley & Sons, 1978), p. 31.

[2]Robert Buxbaum, *Sports for Life* (Boston: Beacon Press, 1979), p. 22.

[3]Pollock, p. 34.

[4]Charles Corbin, *Concepts in Physical Education* 7th ed., (Dubuque, Iowa: Wm. Brown Co., 1990), p. 24.

[5]Pollock, p. 35.

[6]Donald K. Mathews, *The Physiological Basis of Physical Education and Athletics,* 2nd ed. (Philadelphia: W.B. Saunders Co., 1976), p. 280.

[7]David L. Costill, *What Research Tells the Coach About Distance Running* (Washington, D.C.: AAHPER Publications, 1968), p. 5.

[8]Mathews, p. 280.

[9]Barry L. Johnson, *Practical Measurements for Evaluation in Physical Education,* 3rd ed. (Minneapolis: Burgess Publishing Co., 1979), p. 142.

[10]L. Oscai, "Effect of Exercise on Blood Volume," *Journal of Applied Physiology,* XXIV (May, 1968), 622-624.

[11]Mathews, p. 282.

[12]J. L. Boyer, "Exercise Therapy in Hypertensive Men," *Journal of the American Medical Association,* X (March, 1970), 668.

[13]J. L. Boyer, "Effects of Chronic Exercise on Cardiovascular Function," *Physical Fitness Research Digest,* II (1972), 1.

[14]R. J. Shepard, "What Exercise to Prescribe for the Post MI Patient," *The Physician and Sports Medicine,* III (1975), 57.

[15]Corbin, p. 26.

[16]Mathews, p. 16.

[17]Pollock, p. 32.

[18]Mathews, p. 791.

[19]Jean L. Bogert, *Nutrition and Physical Fitness,* 9th ed. (Philadelphia: W.B. Saunders Co., 1973), p. 482.

[20]Pollock, p. 32.

[21]P. Pattengale, "Augmentation of Skeletal Muscle Myoglobin by a Program of Treadmill Running," *American Journal of Physiology,* CCSIII (1967), 783-785.

[22]Jack Wilmore, "Body Composition Changes with a 10-Week Program of Jogging," *Medicine and Science in Sports,* III (1970), 113-117.

[23]Mathews, p. 292.

PSYCHOLOGICAL AND SOCIOLOGICAL ASPECTS OF CARDIOVASCULAR TRAINING

9

The psychological and sociological reasons that individuals choose to participate in aerobic activities are many and varied, from those of companionship, prestige and sense of accomplishment to a sense of control of one's own body. In an age where so many things are complex and beyond the control of the individual, it becomes important for an individual to be able to shape and mold such a complex organism as the human body, even if it is only in a limited manner.[1]

Many individuals in our society today have turned to aerobic training to improve their self-esteem. Society has placed a high value on having a so-called good "physique." Many individuals have felt the need to improve their general appearance in order to gain the admiration of their peers. "The attitudes and feelings of people toward their bodies affect personality development."[2] An individual that perceives himself as being unattractive will frequently show a lack of confidence in himself. Positive physiological changes often occur with continuous aerobic training. Positive changes in an individual's general appearance often enhances his/her self-image.

Many individuals view physical activity as an opportunity for positive emotional release and having fun, thus positively supplementing one's daily living habits.[3] Aerobic training is often characterized as an activity that releases tension and frustration in our complex society.[4] Many philosophers and psychiatrists have done extensive research in this area. Friedrich Nietzche felt in the 19th century that physical activity was a simple outlet for releasing sudden congestion by violent muscular exertion.[5] Nietzche reasoned that anything that did not render permanent harm to the individual would be of benefit. Even in today's so-called "sophisticated" society, there is a need for a socially acceptable outlet to work off an individual's basic instinctive aggressive drives. At this point in society, physical activity seems to be the most socially acceptable method used to work off frustration and anxiety in a way that otherwise might be considered barbaric behavior, i.e., boxing, football, etc.

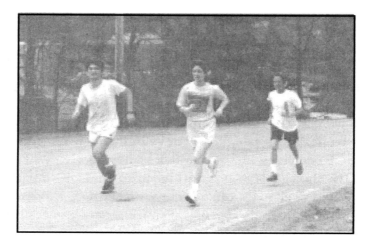

Figure 9.1
Social enjoyment

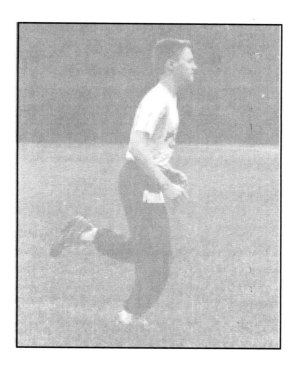

Figure 9.2
Stress reduction

Another psychological issue discussed quite frequently is that of the "runner's high." "Fragmentary but important new information suggests that anxiety and depression are lessened through regular exercise and that the 'natural high' of which so many people speak may have its basis in some hormonal change that takes place as a result of fitness activities."[6] This feeling is appropriately brought into focus when one brings into perspective the fact that when an individual has a lapse in training, the individual will not feel as well as he/she did while participating in continuous training.[7]

Studies on the possible influence of fitness on personality of the individual are still far from complete. Studies have indicted that individuals with high fitness levels are more unconventional, composed, secure, easygoing, emotionally stable, adventurous, and higher in intelligence than those with low fitness levels.[8] The most pronounced personality differences between individuals of high and low fitness levels were those of emotional stability and security. Researchers are still not completely sure whether high levels of training are responsible for these differences, or whether individuals with these personality characteristics are more likely to engage in a fitness program, or if it is a combination of both. Whatever the case may be, just as it takes years to become fit or unfit, significant personality changes are not experienced rapidly.

Aerobic training, as mentioned previously, is excellent for the reduction of anxiety. When highly anxious individuals participate regularly in aerobic training, anxiety is reduced. Individuals with average or low levels of anxiety do not experience a similar reduction as the result of regular training.[9] Research has also indicated that a single session of exercise is more effective in relaxing an individual than a tranquilizer. Exercise is more effective in reducing neuromuscular tension (more complete relief) with no undesirable side effects.[10]

The physical and mental aspects of aerobic training cannot be separated. A proper balance between the physical and mental being of the individual is essential for harmony in the body and optimum performance levels. The positive physiological aspects of aerobic training are many and well worth striving toward. The psychological and sociological benefits vary in that we are all individuals, and what interests one person may not appeal to another person. Whether one's reason for training be for mental release, companionship or self-esteem, one should be consistent and dedicated in his/her training to reap all the mentioned rewards of continuous aerobic training.

NOTES

[1]Robert Buxbaum, *Sports for Life* (Boston: Beacon Press, 1976), p. 6.

[2]Charles A. Bucher, *Foundations of Physical Education,* 10th ed. (St. Louis: C.V. Mosby Co., 1987), p. 191.

[3]Gladys M. Scott, "The Contributions of Physical Activity to Psychological Development," *Research Quarterly,* XXXI, (May, 1960), 307.

[4]John W. Loy, Jr., *Sport, Culture, and Society* (New York: MacMillan Publishing Co., Inc., 1969), p. 76.

[5]D. Levy, *The Complete Works of Friedrich Nietzche* (Edinburgh: Foulis, 1909), p. 291.

[6]Buxbaum, p. 8.

[7]Buxbaum, p. 9.

[8]Brian J. Sharkey, *Physiology of Fitness* (Champaign, Ill.: Human Kinetics Publishers, 1979), p. 201.

[9]W. P. Morgan, "Psychological Effects of Chronic Physical Activity," *Medicine and Science in Sport,* II (Winter, 1970), 213-218.

[10]Hubert A. deVries, "Electromyographic Comparison of Single Doses of Exercise and Meprobromate as to Effects on Muscular Relaxation," *American Journal of Physical Medicine,* LI (1972), 130-141.

MECHANICS OF JOGGING   **10**

The proper mechanics used in jogging are often over-looked because the individual assumes that the ability to jog is inherent in all people. Unfortunately, many individuals have rather poor jogging mechanics and need to be made aware of this fact so that they can correct these flaws in their running form. Realizing that jogging is an activity of high repetition, in that a small flaw in running mechanics is amplified thousands of times in just one training session, one becomes keenly aware of the importance of using the proper running mechanics. At this point, it becomes appropriate for one to study the following proper mechanics of jogging: (1) posture, (2) foot plant, (3) stride, (4) use of arms, (5) breathing, and (6) overall action.

POSTURE

A jogger must maintain proper posture; the body should be in an upright position. Upright means the back is as straight as naturally comfortable, head up, being neither forward nor back of the body line, and the buttocks "tucked in." William J. Bowerman, author of *Jogging,* says, "If in this position, a hypothetical line drawn from the top of your head through the shoulders and hips should be perpendicular, or nearly so."[1] Slouched shoulders, or the typical military posture of throwing back the shoulders and sticking out the chest are not conducive to good jogging mechanics because of the discomfort caused to the lower back and the unnecessary use of energy contracting the back muscles.

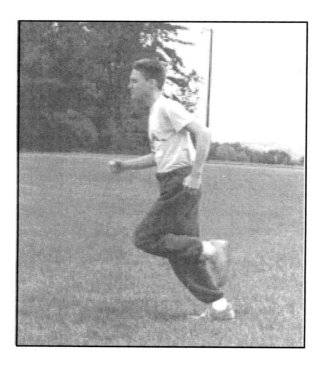

Figure 10.1
Example of slight body lean

Many joggers look at photos that are commonly selected showing the runner will full extension of the driving foot for emphasis on action in running. "Actually, a more valid phase is at mid-stride, when it becomes clear how little lean is present."[2]

FOOT PLANT

The most common mistake made by beginning joggers in relation to foot plant is landing on the ball of the foot first, much the way a sprinter in track would. This type of foot plant is great for speed, but in jogging it puts undue pressure on the calf muscles because of the prolonged contraction of the calf muscles. A more practical and efficient method is the heel-to-toe method of foot plant. In the heel-to-toe method the jogger lands first on the outside portion of the foot and then the heel rocks forward with a slight

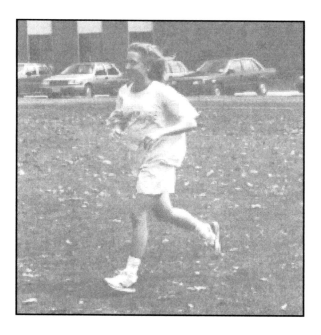

Figure 10.2
Proper foot plant

inward rotation (just enough to prevent a flat footed striking movement, but yet too much rotation can cause knee
problems), and takes off from the ball of the foot. "Hitting
with the heel first cushions the landing, then distributes
the pressure as the foot bends forward."[3] Over prolonged
periods of exercise, the heel-to-toe method conserves more
energy than any other form of foot plant.

The heel-to-toe method was confirmed by Toni Nett in
an extensive study of films of world class long distance
runners. Nett found that all runners made first contact
with the ground on the outside edge of the foot. He also
concluded that first contact is made at the arch between
the heel and the metatarsal bone, as opposed to a sprinter
in track making first contact high on the ball (joints of the
little toe) of the foot.[4]

STRIDE

The most common mistake made by beginning joggers
in relation to leg stride is over-striding. There is a misconception that if one wants to get from one point to another
point, the quickest way is by lengthening the stride.
"Stride length should be approached from the standpoints
of naturalness, and of economy and ease of effort."[5] Over-
striding expends unnecessary amounts of energy, whereas
a shorter stride is much more practical in conservation of
energy to be dispersed over the duration of the exercise.
The most efficient method to cover a distance more quickly
is to shorten the stride length (for the purpose of
conserving energy) and quickening the ratio of stride
cadence. The quickening of stride cadence does not expend
as much energy as lengthening the stride. By the same
token, too short a stride wastes energy by not permitting

the individual to take full advantage of the forward energy generated by the previous muscle contraction.[6] Stride selection generally is an unconscious decision made through trial and error of previous training.

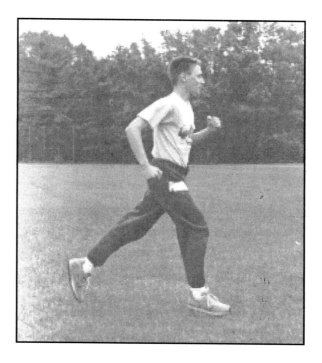

Figure 10.3
Proper stride and arm carriage

USE OF ARMS

Body balance, determination of greater power in leg movements, and freedom from arm fatigue can be greatly aided by the proper use of the arms in jogging. A good general rule of thumb in checking to ensure that the arms are in the proper position is to see if there is approximately a 90 degree angle at the elbows while jogging.[7]The proper angle at the elbows will help to ensure a sound body angle for proper posture while jogging. The proper angle at the elbows will also eliminate undue fatigue that many times will first be experienced in the arms. Factors that cause fatigue in the arms generally center around carrying the arms too high which causes tension in the shoulders and results in clenching the fists. The solution to carrying the arms too high is to relax the shoulders without over-compensating and lowering the arms too much. To alleviate tension in the hands, one should avoid clenching the fists while jogging; touching the tip of the first index finger to the tip of the thumb is an effective way of handling this problem. The arms can also be used to spur the legs on, which in turn speeds up the forward momentum of the individual, thus indicating the significance of the proper movements of the arms.[8]

BREATHING

The correct breathing technique is important so that the diaphragm will be utilized properly. A runner's diaphragm should go down and the belly out when the runner is breathing during a training session. This is not the normal method of breathing for most individuals. By breathing the typical improper way, one stretches the diaphragm in a way that may lead to a stitch (pain in the side that can cause an individual to have to stop and recover before resuming training). How does one learn to use the diaphragm correctly? One method is to lie on the floor with books on one's stomach, and force oneself to breathe so that the books rise.[9] This method should be repeated until this method of breathing becomes natural and second nature. Also, stretching exercises should be done involving the stomach muscles to enhance a more efficient breathing mechanism. Exercises that require breathing out against slight resistance are beneficial because of the necessary contraction of the stomach muscles. Strength and flexibility development in these areas will greatly enhance efficiency in breathing.

In relationship to cadence of breathing patterns, a natural and normal breathing manner should be used. Breathing patterns should be in correspondence to effort needed to sustain training. A good general rule of thumb is that if one becomes so winded that he cannot answer someone who is talking to him, he is pushing himself too hard.

OVERALL ACTION

In considering the coordination of all the proper mechanical aspects of running, such words as rhythm, smoothness, relaxation, and ease of movement must be considered. Proper rhythm in the various mechanical aspects of running will assure a cooperative effort rather than the body working against itself. Smoothness represents movement in such a manner that there is no wasted motion or effort. Every aspect of the body is functioning in a manner that represents maximum return from energy expended. Relaxation is also important in that it represents freedom of movement due to greater range of motion of joints and muscles. Again, running is an activity of high repetition, thus requiring ease of movement to sustain training for prolonged periods of time. Attention must be focused on keeping a vital balance on these and may other factors that contribute to running energy being spent economically. Arthur Lydiard, one of the most successful distance running coaches of all time, warns against not concentrating on the proper mechanics of running. "Don't relax so much that an easy jog becomes a mere amble. While you are moving, keep a constant check on your stride, your balance, the movement of your arms."[10] The significance of the proper mechanics while running are important for reasons varying from injury prevention to less strain during each individual training session.

NOTES

[1]William J. Bowerman, *Jogging* (New York: Charter Books, 1967), p. 25.

[2]Geoffrey Dyson, *The Mechanics of Athletics*, 6th ed. (London: University of London Press, 1974), p. 118.

[3]Bowerman, p. 27.

[4]Toni Nett, "Foot Plant in Running," *Track Technique*, XV (March, 1964), 462.

[5]Kenneth Doherty, *Track and Field Omnibook*, 3rd ed. (Los Altos, Ca.: Track and Field News, 1980), p. 415.

[6]Jack Daniels, *Conditioning for Distance Running* (New York: John Wiley and Sons, 1978), p. 67

[7]Doherty, p. 461.

[8]Dyson, p. 117.

[9]George Sheehan, *Dr. Sheehan on Running* (Mt. View, Ca.: World Publication, 1975), p. 156.

[10]Arthur Lydiard, *Run to the Top* (London: Herbert Jenkins, Ltd., 1962), p. 59.

Environmental Conditions 11

For an individual to be able to embark successfully upon an aerobic training program, he must be able to co-exist successfully with the different environmental conditions he will encounter. For the most part, aerobic training is done outdoors, thus requiring adaptations to weather conditions, appropriate equipment and clothing, differences in running surfaces, terrain differences, and many other variables that need to be taken into consideration in order for optimal training to occur. This unit is concerned with helping the individual maximize a coexistence with the environmental elements encountered in a training regimen.

Training in the Heat

Training in hot climates is a more serious problem than training in cold climates. Exercise increases metabolic heat production which counter-balances heat loss in cold conditions, whereas in a hot climate, metabolism and environment combine to increase significant heat gain in body tissues.[1] The cooling of the body tissues and skin is brought about by the evaporation of sweat. The cooling off of the skin is not the desired end result, rather, it is a by-product of the more important cooling of the internal environment. Continuous training results in a more efficient cooling system because greater volumes of slower moving blood in and close to the skin cause better transfer of heat to the evaporative surfaces.[2]

The ability of an individual to train in a hot environment depends on the following variables:

1. Magnitude of heat
2. Existing humidity
3. Air movement
4. Intensity and duration of training
5. Acclimatization
6. Exposure to the sun
7. Proper clothing
8. Dehydration.

Magnitude of Heat

The higher the temperature, the greater the heat stress placed upon the body. To cool the body, the volume of the circulatory system must increase in proportion to the rise in temperature. To meet this need, the heart rate must increase which depresses cardiac efficiency, putting an additional burden upon the cardiovascular system.[3] The most serious consequence of this inefficiency of the cardiac system is the decrease in blood volume which can lead to a decrease in sweating rate and evaporative cooling. "The decrease in blood volume and evaporative cooling, in turn, causes added circulatory collapse and an excessive rise in rectal temperature."[4]

Existing Humidity

The degree of humidity is of major concern because of its hindrance to the body's efficiency in cooling itself down. As mentioned previously, the body cools itself down during hot conditions by sweating, and if the air is relatively dry, most of the sweat will evaporate and be absorbed by the air thus constituting a continuous cooling cycle. In humid conditions, the air is saturated with water, limiting the evaporation and absorption process and thus causing difficulty in cooling the body.[5] When attempts are made to train to maximum capacity in warm humid conditions, the circulatory process cannot perform both tasks of regulation of body temperature and nutrient delivery to the muscles to optimal levels because of the burden of lessened ability to unload water vapor into already saturated atmospheric conditions.[6] The increased cardiac demand to compensate for body temperature regulation will decrease the efficiency of the individual to train at maximum capacity; thus, it becomes very important to take into consideration not only the outside temperature prior to a training session, but also the amount of humidity in the atmosphere.

Air Movement

The amount of air movement is another critical factor in determining the total stress of training in hot environments. The greater the air movement, the greater the cooling effect. This is a generalization because other factors need to be taken into account such as the quality of the air in regards to humidity and heavy wind conditions which increase the stress of the workload of the individual's training. Also, the direction of the wind has an effect on the cooling process. Running with the wind is not as efficient in terms of cooling effect as running against the wind.[7] When winds are not of a gusty nature, wind velocity and running speed are similar causing a still-air situation when one is running with the wind.

Intensity and Duration of Training

Intensity and duration of the training session also contribute to the total heat stress.

Since the body produces heat as it exercises, the higher the intensity of the exercise and the longer the duration, the greater the resulting heat load and subsequent stress to the body.[8]

Total adaptation to the heat in training will never occur, so heat will always be a major limitation to full-scale training. If the individual must train in the heat, intensity and duration should be modified in proportion to the degree of heat.

Acclimatization

As mentioned in the previous paragraph, it is possible to adapt partially or become acclimated to the heat, but total adaptation never occurs. Because training causes a continuous rise in the body temperature, some degree of heat acclimatization can be attained through training.[9] Short, continuous periods of exposure to heat is the most efficient method of adjusting to training in the heat.[10] It is important to retain as much of the body fluids as possible while training in the heat. This can be accomplished by taking fluids regularly and ensuring a proper intake of salt in the diet to ensure retention of fluids. Excess loss of fluids comes from the blood volume, which will place extra demands on the circulatory system which can lead to long range problems. Individuals respond differently to heat, so adjustments to training in the heat should be made on an individual basis.

Exposure to the Sun

The degree of the sun's radiation will vary with the two most common factors being that of the season of the year and the time of day. During the seasons of the year when hot temperatures are not a problem, training can be done at most any hour of the day. During warmer weather conditions, an effort should be made to train either during the early morning hours when the air is freshest and coolest, or after sunset when the air is driest and there is less direct radiation from the sun.[11] Training in shaded surroundings will lower the stress of training in the heat and also improve the quality of air being breathed. The quality of the training session is directly proportional to the environmental conditions, and heat in extremes such as temperature, humidity or radiation will hinder an individual's performance capabilities.

Proper Clothing

The type of clothing to be worn during training in hot weather conditions is essential to proper adjustments necessary for temperature balance. The following are some guidelines for the type of clothing that should be worn during training in hot weather conditions:[12]

1. Loose-fitting clothing should be worn to expose wetter skin.
2. Tops should be perforated to increase ventilation.

3. Clothing should be light in color to reduce radiation gains.
4. If skin is dry, it should not be wetted.

The wetting of clothing creates a problem in that it hinders the evaporative process by creating a humid "micro-climate" surrounding the individual.

Dehydration

Dehydration is another area in which concern is needed not only because of its negative correlation to physical performance, but also because of its possible seriousness in harming the individual's health. "Physical performance begins to deteriorate when the water deficit exceeds 3 percent of body weight."[13] During exercise of a continuous nature, sweat has less salt than the body's internal fluids, causing the body to be water-poor not salt-poor. Exercising for prolonged periods of time in hot and dry climates may create a need for supplemental salt replacement.[14] To correct this situation, it is advisable to take water and salt in supplemental forms into the body system. Many individuals have trouble taking salt supplements or salt tablets because of irritation to the stomach; with water or carbohydrates such as oranges, apples, etc., the absorption into the body system can be done more effectively and efficiently. It should be noted that habitual heavy users of salt from an early age run a greater risk of developing high blood pressure.[15] Most individuals in our society get adequate amounts of salt in their everyday diet.

Another frequent misconception is that milk causes "cotton mouth" (dryness of mouth) during training sessions. "Dryness of the mouth is due to decreased saliva flow from dehydration of an emotional state."[16] There is no scientific basis for eliminating milk from your diet while you are training. Milk is an excellent source of calcium, essential for children's bones during the growing states. The only reason for elimination of milk from the diet is that the individual has an intolerance to milk, and in this situation would be better off to avoid milk.

The following are three common ailments that occur as a result of over-exposure to the sun for prolonged periods of time:

1. Heat cramps
2. Heat exhaustion
3. Heat stroke.

Heat Cramps

Even well-trained athletes frequently have cramps when they are striving for optimal performance levels in hot environments. The cause of heat cramps is loss of salt through perspiration. Prevention, as well as cure, rests in taking additional salt into one's normal diet. Research has indicated that even under extreme conditions, thirteen to seventeen grams of salt per day will maintain proper electrolyte balance.[17] This special salt requirement represents about one-half ounce and can best be taken by more liberal salting of food. Excessive amounts of salt taken in are excreted but may cause nausea in many individuals, and excessive consumption of salt has a positive correlation with high blood pressure. Salt is important for retention of body fluids. An individual suffering from heat cramps should stop and try to stretch the muscles that are cramping so as to increase circulation and relieve the pain.

Heat Exhaustion

Heat exhaustion occurs when the limitations of the cardiovascular system are exceeded. The symptoms are weak, rapid pulse, with cold skin due to inadequate circulation which will also result in dizziness or fainting.[18] Treatment of a victim of heat exhaustion centers around rest, covering the individual with a blanket to regenerate and retain body heat, and gradually and slowly administering adequate fluids. Inattention to heat cramps and heat exhaustion can lead to irreversible damage to the central nervous system and eventually death.[19] Most individuals will not over-extend themselves to this point, but individuals who are highly motivated and competitive, and subscribe to the old train of thought that water is bad for individuals while training, can extend themselves in hot weather conditions to the point of heat exhaustion. In hot conditions, it becomes important during training sessions to be in tune with one's body, and when it signals the need for fluids, one needs to replenish the body with a water break.

Heat Stroke

Heat stroke occurs as a result of failure of the heat regulatory system. Heat stroke is serious enough to demand immediate medical attention. The symptoms of heat stroke are hot, flushed skin (usually clammy and dry), high body temperature, and unconsciousness.[20] Treatment for heat stroke prior to the arrival of medical attention should consist of trying to lower the body temperature by fanning methods, etc. Immediate treatment is essential not only for survival reasons, but because of the danger of

permanent damage to the hypothalamus and its ability to
regulate body temperature. Many individuals who survive
cases of heat stroke are prone to future heat disorders
because of irreversible damage to the hypothalamus.[21]

TRAINING IN THE COLD

As mentioned earlier in this unit, training in cold
weather conditions presents far fewer problems than training in hot weather conditions. The primary reason that it is
easier to adapt to training in cold weather conditions is
that the body will generate considerable heat while training, and additional clothing can always be worn.[22] To have
a clearer understanding of training in cold weather conditions, one must take a closer look at the following variables
in relationship to training:

1. Limitations
2. Acclimatization
3. Exposure
4. Proper clothing.

Limitations

If the temperature is not low enough to demand excessive amounts of clothing, performance should be enhanced
physiologically.[23] The primary reason for this is the fact
that less blood is needed to be diverted to the skin for cooling purposes. It is important to bear in mind that even in
cold weather conditions many individuals will sweat quite
profusely, resulting in lowered skin temperatures. Accumulation of sweat in clothing and on the skin can result in
substantial heat loss. Another limitation is the fact that fat
is excellent as an insulator against cold, and individuals

who continually participate in aerobic training lower their fat content.[24]

> Other things being equal, the more rotund (endo-morphic) a person, the less surface area he has in rela-tion to volume (mass of tissues); consequently, heat loss occurs at a slower rate than in a person of angular (ec-tomorphic) build.[25]

Thus the round fat person is better able to withstand the cold, and the tall thin person is better able to withstand the heat.

Acclimatization

Continued exposure to cold environments will result in the individual's developing a greater ability to withstand the cold.[26] As mentioned previously, body type will influ-ence the ability of the individual to adapt to cold environ-ments. The body reacts to the cold efficiently by reduction of heat loss and increased metabolism. These physiological characteristics can be aided greatly by continuous aerobic training in cold environments. Psychological factors also contribute greatly to adjustment in cold environments. Hypnosis has been shown to suppress shivering, lower the heart rate, and improve performance significantly during cold exposure at 40 degrees Fahrenheit.[27] This illustrates the value of mental toughness and the experience of par-ticipating in cold environments. This is not to say that a person needs to be hypnotized prior to each training ses-sion, but rather if the mind is prepared properly and espe-cially if it can relate to previous encounters with the cold, efficiency in training will be more likely.

Exposure

As with heat, the degree of humidity plus air movement are important considerations for training in cold weather. The more humid the air, the greater the wind velocity, thus creating greater stress. In dry conditions the individual must be prepared not to overdress so as to be prepared for potential problems with sweating and evaporation which can lead to rapid cooling and chills.[28] Particular attention must be paid to the extremities of the body such as the ears, toes, and fingers because of poor circulation to these areas of the body.

Proper Clothing

In selecting appropriate clothing for training in cold environments, protection against the elements is obviously important, but wearing clothing that allows the proper flow of moist air from the body is also of great importance. The whole idea of protection against the cold is defeated if the type of clothing used traps the moisture between itself and the body, causing a further chilling effect. Wool and cotton are the best materials for appropriate clothing for training in the cold.[29] Warmup suits that do not have efficient evaporative qualities (such as rubber-lined suits) should be avoided. Also, any metal jewelry or watch bands that are exposed to freezing temperatures should be avoided because of high conduction potentials. For protection of the extremities, usually wool caps and mittens will suffice. The feet have less trouble keeping warm, but appropriate socks are important as a precautionary measure.[30]

AIR POLLUTION

Air pollution has become a widespread problem in our society and is no longer restricted to heavily populated metropolitan areas. Carbon monoxide is the largest contributor to the air pollution problem in society. Carbon monoxide has a much greater attraction to hemoglobin than oxygen.[31] Most oxygen is transported through the blood by hemoglobin. Thus, high concentrations of carbon monoxide will have a significantly negative effect on an individual's training capacity. Since automobiles release significant levels of carbon monoxide, caution is advised when one is training along heavily traveled roads. Training in areas such as parks is safer because of a less polluted environment, and it also reduces the risk of traffic problems.

TRAINING AT HIGH ALTITUDES

The higher the altitude in which an individual is training, the less the atmospheric pressure. The less the pressure, the harder it is to drive oxygen into the blood. This necessitates the individual's breathing more air to attempt to get the same number of molecules of oxygen. This increased effort of the respiratory muscles to consume more oxygen results in a lowered efficiency in the body's training capacity.[32] The effect of decreased efficiency is in proportion to the altitude in which the individual is training. At 3,000 feet, an individual will lose five percent of aerobic capacity, and as much as fifteen percent at 6,500 feet.[33] For individuals not used to training at higher altitudes, it is advisable to lessen the intensity of training sessions and to start out at a slower pace than usual to avoid building up an immediate oxygen debt.

TERRAIN

Hill Running

Training on hilly terrain can be an effective method of increasing the intensity of the training session because of the fact that maintaining the same pace while running uphill increases the energy demand. There are some potential hazards that need to be considered in hill training. Hill training requires the use of fast, white muscle fibers, which are generally untrained in distance runners. White muscle fibers can lead to muscle fatigue and increased risk of potential injury.[34] Hill training also is very strenuous on tendons, ligaments, and joints of the leg muscles. Because of the strain to the legs, hill training requires recovery after a training session and should not be used more than two to three times a week. Because of the fatigue and strain to the leg muscles as a result of hill running, individuals just getting started in an aerobics program or at low levels of fitness should probably either avoid hill running or do very little hill running.

The mechanics of hill running are different from running on level terrain. It is necessary to shorten the stride slightly in order to maintain the center of gravity over the drive leg.[35] Also, it is important to exaggerate one's forward lean, and the arms need to be pumped harder in a jabbing style much like a boxer in order to attack the hill and direct the force up the hill. Running into the wind is similar to the amount of resistance encountered in running hills, and the running mechanics should be similar. In running downhill, one should lengthen the stride to maintain the center of gravity slightly in front of the drive leg. It is important to note that any time one lengthens the stride, greater force is generated and must be absorbed by the legs, knees, and hips.[36] Also, the muscle groups are not used to being extended in this manner, and this often causes additional strain.

Different Types of Surfaces

Different types of surfaces individuals train on can be classified into two categories: hard and soft. Hard surfaces include asphalt, concrete, and many running tracks of either clay composition or asphalt composition. Soft surfaces include grass or types of turf that have a degree of give to them to cushion the blow of the foot striking the surface. There are advantages and disadvantages to training on both types of surfaces.

Running on concrete sidewalks produces more shock which requires cushioning by the iliotibial tract than running on grass or even asphalt.[37] The iliotibial tract stabilizes the knee between the femur and the tibia, the bones adjoining at the knee from opposite directions.[38] Running on hard surfaces also increases the force to the legs, and causes excessive use of foot flexor muscles which can lead to pain and discomfort to the legs and eventually a number of stress-related injuries such as shin splints.[39] When running on roads, one should be careful to avoid roads that are noticeably crowned for water run-off. This crown causes the foot closest to the crowned part of the road to pronate (turn inward), causing stress to both foot and knee.[40] Hard surfaces are popular to train on in many instances because they are faster than soft surfaces. In many instances, it is much easier to find roads that are appropriate for training for prolonged periods of time as opposed to finding soft surfaces such as a park. There is also a significantly reduced chance of ankle injury when one is training on hard surfaces as opposed to soft surfaces.[41]

Soft surfaces are beneficial for protection against overuse injuries caused by the highly repetitious nature of running. Softer surfaces such as grass tend to have more shock-absorbing potential than hard surfaces, thus being easier on the legs and knees. Potential hazards of jogging on softer surfaces include ankle injuries because of the nature of uneven terrain, chuck-holes, etc. Running on grass also requires more energy expenditure because of the absorbing potential of grass.

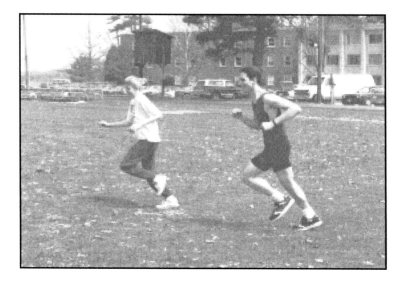

Figure 11.1
Running on grass

Shoes

Because of the highly repetitious nature of jogging, the proper footwear is extremely important. Buying the most expensive model of shoe does not necessarily guarantee the proper shoe for your specific needs. No one specific shoe has been manufactured that meets the footwear needs of everyone. Thus, it is vital to try on different shoes to judge what shoe best fits one's personal needs. Being careful not to lace the shoes too tightly and checking to see if the tongue of the shoe is padded so as not to rub the top portion of the foot unnecessarily is also important. The shoe should be constructed of a material that breathes well, to prevent excess accumulation of perspiration in the

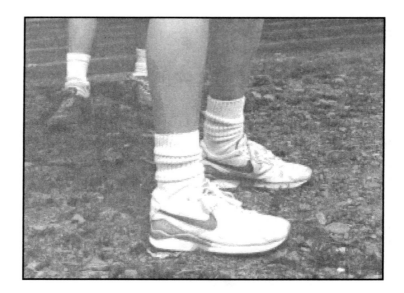

Figure 11.2
Example of quality running shoes

shoe. A wider heel and a softer shoe cushion dampens the shock transmitted from the running surface.[42] There are a number of popular running magazines on the market that rate running shoes. The objectivity of the rating is suspect because some of the rated shoes advertise in the magazine, and it is questionable whether or not the magazine would rate them low if it were appropriate to do so. The ratings, if used properly, can clue the individual into possibly three or four pairs of shoes that merit consideration. Again, realizing that all are individuals and needs differ, one should try on the different brands of shoes and decide which of the rated shoes best fits his/her needs.

THINGS RESEARCH DOES NOT TELL YOU ABOUT JOGGING

The following information is based on practical application of many years of jogging. The material that I will be sharing is a culmination of personal experience and countless conversations with many joggers who have learned these lessons, many by trial-and-error. It is the author's hope that by sharing this information, that you will avoid many of the pitfalls that normally a novice in this area would experience.

Running in the City

The biggest challenge that a jogger faces when attempting to run in an urban environment is trying to avoid a traffic signal light every block. The best way to avoid this dilemma is to look for sections of the city where you can jog for extended distances without encountering signal lights. Some examples of such areas might include parks, river banks, industrial parks, bridges, etc.

Where do you jog in a strange city?

A significant challenge for the jogger who does a significant amount of traveling is finding a place to jog in an unfamiliar city. Many hotels furnish maps that show jogging loops of differing distances. If your hotel does not furnish this information, the desk clerk often will be a good source of information for creating your own jogging course. Another way of gaining insight as to where to jog is to call the local YMCA or health Spa. They may even have specific times when members gather together to do their daily run.

What do you do with your keys?

Very few joggers want to carry their keys with them on their run. One way of eliminating this problem is to take your door key and tie it into the top laces of your running shoes. This will only take a minute to do, but will effectively free your hands so that during the run you can utilize the proper running form. Many athletic stores sell vinyl cases that slip onto shoe laces.

Jogging against traffic

When jogging on the roads, it is important to jog against the flow of traffic. This will allow you to see oncoming traffic and make any adjustments necessary for safety reasons. Most motorists will go out of their way to avoid a dangerous situation. But, it is better to exercise extra caution on your part than to challenge a rude driver in an automobile.

Identification

When going out for a jog, it is a good idea to have some type of identification in case of emergency. This also can be carried in your case that carries your door key. Another technique utilized quite frequently by joggers to wear some type of personalized running gear.

Running at Night

It is not advisable to jog after dark. It is also dangerous during that thirty-minute period before evening or the start of the morning because of decreased visibility for drivers. If you decide to jog in the evening hours, it is important to wear light colored clothing that can be more easily seen by motorists. There are a number of reflective running gear items (vest, reflective tape to place on running attire, reflective pieces built into running shoes) that can be bought at most athletic stores.

Dogs

One of the most annoying problems that joggers often face is the dog that does not want to allow you to jog in front of its property. Many dogs will just want to follow you for a short distance (a little bit of friendly attention can go a long way). If this is not the case, it is probably advisable to stop until the dog goes away or the owner convinces the dog to retreat. In rural areas you will normally find that dogs are trained not to cross the street for safety reasons. So if you know this is the case, jogging on the other side of the street may prove to be a successful strategy.

Why don't you act your age!

Many individuals in our society are not convinced that jogging is something adults (especially senior adults) should be doing. There are many reasons for this attitude. The significance should not be one of the reasons why people in our society feel this way, but that jogging is a personal activity that brings joy and satisfaction to the individual. Besides, who really wants to grow up?

So you want to enter your first 10K race!

Many joggers will progress to the point that they want to enter their first road race. Entering a race can provide a good assessment of the individual's conditioning level. Some cautions for an individual entering his first race:

1. Do not try to compete against other runners—stay within your own limitations
2. Do some type of pace training prior to the race so that you will have a general idea of the pace that you can comfortably run
3. Your first race can be an emotional experience, be careful not to get too excited and go-out too fast in the first part of the race
4. Be careful to hold back a little on your pace the first half of the race; it is better to finish strong than to be suffering at the completion of the race

5. Know the course so that you can judge mile intervals
6. If it is a 10K race or longer, be sure to take in ample quantities of fluids during the race.

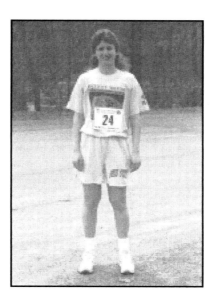

Figure 11.3
Ready for that first race

Being around other joggers at a race can be a positive time of affirmation. The key is to run within your limitations and not to be hard on yourself if you do not measure up to the expectations of others.

UV RAYS: THE BASIC FACTS

"The sun's rays are a major source of vitamin D and help the body's systems acquire much needed calcium for building healthy bones. "[43] Sadly many people in our culture spend large amounts of time in the sun and do not take the necessary precautions to prevent a wide variety of problems. The most common of these problems is the simple attempt to increase ones tan that progresses to the point of sunburn. This comes from the process of the ultraviolet rays from the sun penetrating the skin and stimulating cells containing a brownish pigment called melanin.[44] People with dark skins have a higher amount of melanin and thus have a greater protection from ultraviolet rays. Fair skinned individuals and blondes have less melanin and therefore burn more quickly. Skin damage from overexposure to these rays over the years is cumulative and cannot be reversed. Most serious and lasting damage occurs before the age of 18.

Some of the more serious problems associated with overexposure to ultraviolet rays include:

1. Cancer — The most common being melanoma which accounts for 73% of deaths from skin cancer.
2. Premature aging of skin — including wrinkles and skin that becomes leathery in appearance.
3. Sunlight and allergic reactions — including severe burn or skin eruptions.
4. Eye damage — including corneal sunburn and growths of the surface of the eyes that can be prevented by the use of sunglasses that block 99% –100% of UVA radiation. [45]

A common sense approach would tell an individual to do what our friends from Australia call "slip, slop, slap (slip on a shirt, slop on a hat, and slap on some sunscreen). Also being aware of being out at different times of the day (best hours being before 10:00 a.m. and after 4:00 p.m.) to exercise. Being aware of the fact that the closer you are to the equator, the more intense the ultraviolet rays will be. Also the higher the elevation, the less protection you will have because the air and cloud cover are less.

Sun Screens

Sun screens can be effective protection against ultraviolet rays because they absorb and scatter ultraviolet rays. They utilize a numerical rating system to indicate the specific amount of protection they offer. The numbers, known as Sun Protection Factors (SPF), are listed on the product. The higher the SPF number, the greater the protection. If applied properly, your skin will get the equivalent of one minute of UVB rays for each 15 minutes you spend in the sun. [46]

Clothing for Sun Protection

For many years fair skinned people have utilized the approach of wearing long pants and long sleeve shirts for optimum protection. Fabrics that have a tighter weave or knit, denser, and in darker colors provide better protection. [47] These types of fabrics tend to be more hot and less comfortable to wear. There are numerous companies that presently market UV resistant clothing that is very comfortable to wear and offers great protection. These companies also market a wide variety of running hats that are excellent for providing additional protection for the individual.

NOTES

[1]Hubert deVries, *Physiology of Exercise* (Dubuque, Iowa: W. C. Brown Co., 1980), p. 505.

[2]deVries, p. 505.

[3]deVries, p. 506.

[4]Donald K. Mathews, *The Physiological Basis of Physical Education and Athletics,* 2nd ed. (Philadelphia: W.B. Saunders Co., 1976), p. 115.

[5]Michael L. Pollock, *Health and Fitness Through Physical Activity* (New York: John Wiley and Sons, 1978), p. 237.

[6]David Costill, *What Research Tells the Coach About Distance Running* (Washington, D.C.: AAHPER Publications, 1968), p. 42.

[7]Jack Daniels, *Conditioning for Distance Running* (New York: John Wiley and Sons, 1978), p. 34.

[8]Pollock, p. 238.

[9]N. B. Strydom, "Acclimatization to Humid Heat and the Role of Physical Conditioning," *Journal of Applied Physiology,* XXXI (March, 1966), 636-642.

[10]Costill, p. 44.

[11]Daniels, p. 36.

[12]Costill, p. 44.

[13]L. Jean Bogert, *Nutrition and Physical Fitness,* 9th ed. (Philadelphia: W.B. Saunders Co., 1973), p. 488.

[14]Robert Buxbaum, *Sports for Life* (Boston: Beacon Press, 1979), p. 60.

[15]Buxbaum, p. 57.

[16]Charles Corbin, *Concepts in Physical Education* 7th ed., (Dubuque, Iowa: W. C. Brown Co., 1990), p. 226.

[17]H. L. Taylor, "The Effect of Sodium Chloride Intake on the Work Performance of Man During Exposure to Dry Heat and

Experimental Heat Exhaustion," *American Journal of Physiology,* CXL (1943), 439-451.

[18]Hubert A. deVries, *Physiology of Exercise* (Dubuque, Iowa: Wm. Brown Co., 1980), p. 508.

[19]Donald K. Mathews, *The Physiological Basis of Physical Education and Athletics,* 2nd ed. (Philadelphia: W. B. Saunders Co., 1976), p. 116.

[20]deVries, p. 509.

[21]Mathews, p. 116.

[22]Pollock, p. 238.

[23]Jack Daniels, *Conditioning for Distance Running* (New York: John Wiley & Sons, 1978), p. 37.

[24]Costill, p. 45.

[25]deVries, p. 512.

[26]deVries, p. 503.

[27]A. T. Kissen, "Modification of Thermoregulatory Responses to Cold by Hypnosis," *Journal of Applied Physiology,* XIX (November, 1964), 1043-1050.

[28]Pollock, p. 239.

[29]Daniels, p. 36.

[30]Daniels, p. 37.

[31]Pollock, p. 239.

[32]deVries, p. 515.

[33]P. O. Astrand, "Physiological Aspects of Cross-Country Skiing at High Altitudes," *Journal of Sports Medicine and Physical Fitness,* III (1963), 51-52.

[34]Daniels, p. 64.

[35]Daniels, p. 67.

[36]Gerald Mayfield, "Runner's Knee," *Medicine Sport,* XII (1978), 138.

[37]Mayfield, p. 137.

[38]Katharine F. Wells, *Kinesiology,* 6th ed. (Philadelphia: W. B. Saunders Co., 1976), p. 165.

[39]Daphne Benas, "Shin Splints," *Medicine Sport,* XII (1978), 134.

[40]Robert M. Parks, "Injuries of the Endurance Athlete," *Medicine Sport,* XII (1978), 145.

[41]Parks, p. 150.

[42]Mayfield, p. 138.

[43] Perin, Angela. (2005, January). Sun Expsoure & UV Rays: The Basic Facts, EzineArticles

[44] Sun Safety: http://www.medicalcenter.osu.edu/patient care/healthinformation/otherhelathtopics/Non-Traumatic Emercencies/PreventingUnintentionalln4624/SunSafety/

[45] Skin Cancer Fact Sheet: http://www.aad.org/aad/ Newsroom/2005+Skin+Cancer+Fact+Sheet.htm

[46] Facts about Sunscreens: http://www. Aad.org/public/ News/DermInfo/DInfoSunscreenFAQ.htm

[47] Sun Protective Clothing: http://www.ftc.gov/bcp/ conline/pubs/alerts/sunalrt.htm

INJURY PREVENTION AND CARE   12

Because of the tremendous force of repetitive heel and foot contact that must be dissipated throughout the lower limbs and spine, almost all injuries that can be associated with aerobic training arise in the lower extremities.[1] The key to prevention of running injuries lies in how well the athlete handles the stress of continuous ground reactive force to the lower extremities. This involves eliminating musculoskeletal imbalances or inadequacies. Because of the repetitive nature of running, (the foot strikes the ground over 5,000 times during a one-hour period), these types of injuries are generally classified as overuse injuries.[2]

Some of the more common overuse injuries reported in runners are knee-related complaints, 25%; shin splints, 12%; Achilles tendonitis, 20%; and foot-related problems, 15%; a general observation also shows that women have more hip pain than men.[3] The greater incidence of hip pain in women centers around the fact that women have a wider pelvis than men and tend to have a greater swaying or crossover effect in the pelvis, causing greater incidence of pain occurrence because of the strain to the iliotibial band. As mentioned in the previous paragraph, injuries occur because of imbalances or inadequacies. The repetitive nature of running will increase the likelihood and severity of injury if the imbalance or inadequacy is present and the individual continues to train without controlling the problem in one way or another. This explains the reason why some individuals can train long and hard and remain basically injury free, while other individuals with defects in technique or musculoskeletal build become injured quite frequently. The learning of how to train injury free is important because continual training and stress used the correct way lead to the ultimate in fitness.[4]

Because a slight variation from the proper mechanics of running can produce such negative results, training patterns and running form should frequently be analyzed to assure all components are contributing to the well-being of the individual. Most individuals need an injury or two to remind them that their bodies are stressed and they need to be aware of the body's tolerance to training and its limitations. A problem that is quite frequent is that the muscles worked by continual training become too tight and overdeveloped while their antagonist (opposite working muscle group) muscles do not have the opportunity to develop proportionally. It is recommended that the antagonist muscles should have 60% the strength of the primary muscle groups.[5] Prevention for this centers around strength development and flexibility development so as to have the proper balance between the two muscle groups. This can be accomplished through a proper balance between ballistic stretching exercises and static stretching exercises along with a good balanced weight-lifting program that does not limit flexibility.

OVERUSE INJURIES

As mentioned previously, overuse injuries are frequent in aerobic training because of the repetitive nature of running. Overuse injuries occur when abnormal amounts of stress are placed upon the body by improper technique or genetic disorders. There are many different types of over-use injuries, but research, as indicated on the previous page, shows the following injuries are most frequent and prevention and care need to be exercised:

1. Achilles tendonitis
2. Runner's knee
3. Shin splints
4. Stress fractures
5. Morton's Foot.

Achilles Tendonitis

"Achilles tendonitis is an inflammation or swelling of the Achilles tendon near its point of insertion in the back of the heel bone."[6] The Achilles tendon is a very strong tendon running from the calf to the back of the heel. The Achilles Tendon's function is to bring the foot down during the forward body progression phase of running. The primary symptoms of Achilles tendonitis are tightness and pain in the very back of the ankle region. The primary cause of Achilles tendonitis is excessive side-to-side motion of the heel bone which causes a strain to the Achilles tendon, resulting in swelling and pain. Tightness in the calf muscles because of genetic reasons, poor running technique, or lack of proper conditioning, may place additional stress on the Achilles tendon by increasing the tension.

Achilles tendonitis frequently begins as a tightness sensation which will only worsen with continued running. Running on soft surfaces will decrease the discomfort, but the most effective treatment is reducing the swelling with ice and decreasing training proportions until complete recovery is established. It is also important to avoid hill running because of the obvious stress to the Achilles tendon. Stabilization of the heel to avoid excessive motion is important for proper treatment. This can be accomplished by utilizing proper taping techniques and heel supports. A felt heel lift of $\frac{1}{8}$ to $\frac{1}{4}$ inch can effectively decrease the strain on the Achilles tendon.[7] It is important to realize that Achilles tendonitis is the type of injury that will only worsen if training is not modified and can progress to the stage of being a very serious and disabling injury. When this type of problem becomes frequent, medical advice should be sought.

Runner's Knee

Runner's knee is referred to as the inflammation of the cartilage behind the patella or knee cap due to erosion or irritation. "Essentially, the patella becomes fissured (separated), develops changes in the hyaline cartilage, the smooth shiny surface underneath becomes soft and finally degenerative arthritis results."[8] An early symptom is pain from under the knee cap, especially when one is running downhill or walking upstairs.[9] The most common cause of knee problems is excessive pronation (foot turning inward excessively) of the foot which causes internal rotation of the knee. Another frequent cause of knee problems is increasing training too rapidly, thereby not giving the body a chance to adequately adapt to increased intensity of the training sessions.

In considering the area of prevention for knee problems, proper conditioning and dealing with inherent musculoskeletal weaknesses must be dealt with. When vigorous training is attempted without proper preparation, the muscles most often will be too weak to effectively stabilize the knee.[10] This will place excessive stress on muscle tendons and ligaments resulting in fatigue and damage to soft tissue structures. Musculoskeletal weaknesses in the feet contribute to faulty foot mechanics which often lead to knee problems. Because of the additional strain to the ligaments and tendons, stability of the joints of the knee is decreased. Many times an orthotic insert to the shoe will correct any inherent weakness of the foot. A cast of the neutral position of the foot (position which is considered proper mechanically) is made and worn during the training session to assure proper foot placement. Treatment for runner's knee should be directed at maintaining the knee cap in proper alignment to minimize irritation. Reduction in quantity of training in addition to avoiding hills is essential when recovering or rehabilitating knee problems. When swelling is present, ice should be applied both before and after the training session.[11] Since the quadricep muscles stabilize the knee, exercises that will strengthen this group of muscles will be beneficial. Static stretching exercises should be used exclusively until the pain subsides. As mentioned in the previous unit, running on roads that are noticeably crowned should be avoided as well as continually running around a track in the same direction, thus putting excessive stress on the inside leg.

⌐ *Shin Splints*

Shin splints refer to an overuse injury in which the leg muscles are pulled away from the bony attachment on the tibia.[12] This pulling away of the muscle from the bone causes pain in the middle of the leg on the inside portion of the tibia (bone in shin portion of leg.)[13] The cause of shin splints is not known, but contributing factors are dropped

arches, pulled muscles, running on toes before an individual is in shape, inflammation, muscle spasms, strained
muscles, inadequate blood supply to muscles in this area,
and training excessively on hard surfaces.[14] Shin splints
are thought to be a result of muscular overuse because of
genetic foot imbalance or improper running mechanics
which causes abnormal stress and fatigue to the muscles in
the shin area, thus causing pain and inflammation.

Prevention of shin splints includes proper conditioning
prior to increasing intensity and duration of training,
especially if training is going to be done on hard surfaces
(hard surfaces should be avoided if possible). Taping under the arches for support, and taping directly to the shins
to prevent muscle tears, can be effective preventive measures. Treatment for shin splints is rest. Shin splints cannot
be "run out" under any circumstances. Individuals that try
to "run out" shin splints will have s false sense of cure.
This method of treatment leads to the development of scar
tissue and a form of bone growth that cannot be absorbed
or worked out of the body.[15] To prevent further swelling
and reduce pain, ice should be applied prior to and immediately following each training session. Training sessions
should be limited to tolerance level of an individual and
not be pushed beyond those limits. If the above-mentioned
methods of treatment are not successful in relieving the
pain, rest from training should be imposed for at least a
couple of weeks. If shin splints are not treated properly,
the following sequence will occur frequently:

1. Pain
2. Involuntary disuse
3. Muscle atrophy
4. Stress overload
5. Muscle fatigue

6. Loss of shock absorption
7. Structural stress to bone
8. Stress fracture.[16]

The importance of immediate and appropriate treatment for shin splints is essential because of the potential negative effects that go along with neglect of this overuse injury.

Stress Fractures

Stress fractures are small breaks which occur in bones that are subjected to continuous trauma.[17] Stress fractures related to aerobic training are frequently experienced in the metatarsals (bones responsible for movement of toes), although it is not uncommon to experience stress fractures in the heel bone or leg bones. Metatarsal stress fractures are a result of one metatarsal bearing a disproportionate amount of weight during the foot plant of the running mechanics. This weight imbalance causes many problems such as excessive pronation of the foot and other negative effects which can lead to stress fractures of the metatarsal bones. Stress fractures of the heel bone and leg bones are associated with improper heel plant causing excessive force to the heel. Treatment for stress fractures includes rest to allow the breaks in the bones the opportunity to heal. Functional orthoses are excellent for stabilizing the metatarsals and distributing the weight more evenly, but stress fractures in the heel and leg bones are due to body impact at heel contact: thus this syndrome will not respond to orthotics.[18] Proper running mechanics in regard to heel contact with the ground, along with shoes that have good heel support, and training on soft surfaces will help avoid potential problems and help the rehabilitation process.

Morton's Foot

Morton's foot is a hereditary deformity in which the individual has a shortened first toe and a long second toe. The shortened first toe is a result of an abnormally short first metatarsal bone which is extremely hypermobile at its base.[19] The long second toe is a result of an abnormally long second metatarsal bone. This type of foot places an unproportionate weight burden on the second metatarsal bone, causing it to bear more than its share of weight. "This allows the foot to become hypermobile, flatten, or pronate."[20] This hypermobility of the foot forces an adaptation by either bearing most of the weight on the head of the second metatarsal bone, leading to a potential stress fracture; or pronating the foot, which can lead to leg stress, fractures, runner's knee and severe hip pain.[21]

Proper diagnosis is essential in considering whether an individual has Morton's Foot. A long second toe does not always mean that an individual has Morton's Foot. Many individuals have a long second toe but have no difficulty training rigorously. Individuals that suspect they may have Morton's Foot should have x-rays taken to determine the relationships of the metatarsal bones.[22] The key to treatment of Morton's Foot is the taking of proper preventive measures to ensure the least possible force being generated to the metatarsal bones while training. This can best be accomplished by the proper selection of appropriate footwear that cushions the shock while running and gives additional protection to the metatarsal heads. A heavier, well-padded pair of training shoes is essential for cushioning the shock of the continual nature of training. Periodically, one should check the shoes to see that there is not excessive wear under the ball of the foot and on the outside of the heel; abnormal amounts of stress being placed on metatarsals can lead to many stress-related injuries. An insole worn with a well-padded pair of training shoes will work very efficiently in cushioning the shock and protecting the metatarsal bones. Homemade inserts adjusting for the differences needed to compensate for the longer second toe can be very effective. In severe cases of Morton's Foot, a rigid orthotic with an extension for adaptation for the longer second toe may be necessary. Because a recent study states that 30% of individuals with lower leg injuries have Morton's Foot, proper prevention and care is essential to eliminate unnecessary injuries related to Morton's Foot.[23]

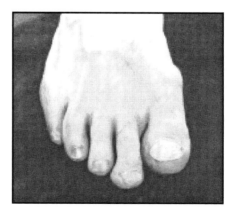

Figure 12.1
Possible Morton's foot

MINOR INJURIES

In relationship to aerobic training, overuse injuries are very common in individuals who do not stay in tune with their bodies when the body communicates excessive amounts of stress to the individual. Yet with proper preventive and care measures, one can eliminate or lessen the severity of overuse injuries, thus enabling more fruitful training. However, overuse injuries are not the only type of injuries with which individuals participating in aerobic training need to concern themselves. There are many other types of injuries, less severe in nature, that may not incapacitate the individual from training, but can be very annoying and in many cases disturb normal training patterns. Some of the more common injuries that warrant discussion are the following:

1. Ankle sprains
2. Heel spurs
3. Blisters
4. Athlete's foot
5. Calluses
6. Ingrown toenails.

Ankle Sprains

A sprain is the result of a joint injury of the ligaments resulting from deformation or excessive motion of the joint.[24] Excessive movement of the ligaments frequently results in tearing, causing hemorrhage beneath the skin, disability, and pain. Most frequently this occurs to the outer side of the ankle, where it is called an eversion sprain, rather than to the inside of the ankle, where it is called an inversion type of sprain.[25]

To understand more fully the cause and prevention of ankle sprains, it is important to understand the makeup of the ankle. The ankle is made up of three bones, the tibia and fibula, both from the lower leg, and the talus, which is from the foot. The ankle is considered to be a saddle-type joint because of the way the three bones converge together resembling a saddle with the body being able to pivot over it.[26] Being a joint, it must have proper stability and alignment. Ligaments and tendons are primarily responsible for this much-needed stability of the ankle joint. The ligaments of the ankle restrict excessive foot inversion or eversion. Damage to the ligaments can minimize efficiency of support and mobility characteristics of the ankle, thus making the ankle more susceptible to injury. Tendons cross the ankle on both sides, thus providing stability. One set of tendons pulls the foot into inversion, while another set of tendons pulls the foot into eversion. The counter-reaction causes a neutralizing effect, thus enhancing stability.[27]

Ankle joints that are relatively stiff and lacking in flexibility are more susceptible to sprains.[28] Thus, the best prevention of ankle sprains involves stretching and flexibility exercises that maintain full motion about the joints. This is especially important in rehabilitation circumstances to increase flexibility and strength development in order to avoid reoccurrence. As mentioned previously, soft surfaces are excellent for prevention of many overuse injuries, but for a runner with ankle problems there is a significantly greater risk of ankle injury while training on soft surfaces. Treatment of an ankle sprain should include the following precautionary measures. First, the shoe and sock should be removed so as not to stimulate any further swelling.

Elevation of the ankle is also important to help minimize potential swelling. Ice should be wrapped around the ankle region.[29] The ice constricts the blood vessels to retard swelling and also acts as an anesthetic in reducing pain.[30] No weight should be placed upon the ankle until it has been examined.

Heel Spurs

Heel spurs are caused initially by persistent irritation that induces the foot to develop a fluid-filled sac under the skin near the bone. The sac frequently becomes harder and fibrous in nature as irritation continues until it finally develops into a growth on the bone in the area of the heel.[31] These small sacs are called bursaes, and function as shock absorbers. When the bursae becomes inflamed and enlarged, the heel becomes very timid and less effective in handling the repetitive stress of running. This condition frequently starts out as an area of redness or blister formation at the back of the heel, with the primary cause being excessive pronation of the foot.

To prevent heel spurs, one should wear a functional orthotic that will effectively prevent abnormal heel motion, the major cause of heel spurs. Avoiding hill running is also very important when early symptoms occur, in addition to wearing shoes with a good heel lift. Treatment for heel spurs involves ice therapy for relief of inflammation. Steroid injections can be beneficial but usually require the individual to stop running to allow the bursae to heal properly.[32] A piece of felt or foam with the center cut out as a cushion to relive pressure on this area can be effective. A heel spur injury is not the type of injury that can be ignored. Because of the location near the Achilles tendon and the possibility of irritation to this tendon, proper treatment is essential. Reduction of the stress or stopping of training is essential until the problem is corrected because severe cases of heel spurs require surgical removal and generally lead to other complications.

Blisters

"A blister is the separation of the outer layer of skin from the inner layer with the intervening space becoming filled with a watery substance or blood.[33] Blisters most frequently occur at sites of bony prominences such as around the little toe. The causes are many and varied, but frequently involve friction and pinching by either poorly fitted shoes or wrinkled socks. Dirty socks and poor quality shoes are also suspect in regard to problems with blisters. To prevent blisters, one should make sure that shoes and socks fit properly, that socks are clean and that poor quality shoes are discarded. Treatment for blisters should involve covering the affected area with a sterile pad and keeping the area as clean as possible.[34] Rehabilitation can also be aided by the use of antiseptics. There is some controversy over whether to open a blister. If a blister is opened, the needle used must be sterilized to prevent possible contamination. Also, the blister should be covered with a dry sterile pad after it is opened. If a blister is not opened, it will frequently harden into a callus or open on its own. If an individual chooses not to open a blister, he/she should place a dry sterile pad on the blister so if the blister opens there is no danger of infection.

Athlete's Foot

Athlete's foot is a chronic scaly condition with redness and itching between the toes, and in some extreme cases, on the bottom of the foot.(The cause of athlete's foot is excessive moisture in the area of the foot. Frequently careless drying habits, the use of moist and moldy sweat socks, and walking barefoot around the shower room collecting excessive amounts of moisture will cause athlete's foot. Since athlete's foot is a fungus, it thrives on a warm, moist environment such as the area between the toes. This fungus growth must be combated, or the itching and peeling of the skin between the toes and the bottoms of the feet can sideline an individual for as long as four to six weeks.[35]

Prevention of athlete's foot involves proper airing and drying of athletic clothing, use of clean socks, and daily application of foot powder. It also involves proper washing of feet and toes daily, and special attention should be given to drying between the toes after bathing. Clean feet and clean, dry socks are the most efficient methods of prevention and treatment of athlete's foot. Once an individual experiences athlete's foot, constant observation is necessary to prevent future occurrences of this problem.

Calluses

"A callus is a thickened, horny layer of skin which most frequently occurs under the joints of the toes or on the heel of the foot."[36] A callus is most frequently caused by poorly-fitted shoes, dropped arches, or a portion of the foot carrying more than its share of weight. Prevention of a callus can be accomplished by the use of skin tougheners, metatarsal pads, and wearing properly fitted shoes. Taping of the arches can relieve tension and evenly distribute weight. This can be accomplished by placing a strip of two-inch tape under the middle of the arch, gently lifting upward and snugly attaching it on top of the foot.[37]

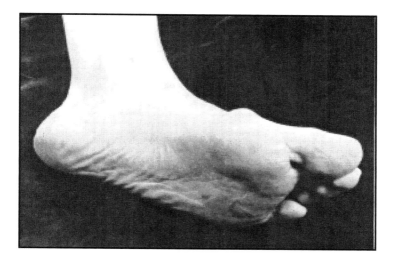

Figure 12.2
Calluses

A callus is not the type of injury that will hinder an individual's training patterns. Through the use of proper taping techniques and pads, a callus becomes more of a nuisance than a disabling type of injury; however, a callus can be serious if it is caused by weight distribution imbalance which can lead to severe foot and leg problems. Treatment of a callus primarily involves soaking the foot in hot water then filing off the loose portion of skin with a callus file or piece of sandpaper.

Ingrown Toenail

"An ingrown toenail is an overlapping of the nail by the adjacent tissue and is often attended by painful ulceration."[38] The most frequent cause of ingrown toenails is rounding off the toenail instead of cutting it straight across, thus creating a downward pressure on the nail and an upward and inward pressure of the flesh. This can also be attributed to improperly fitted shoes or socks. Prevention of ingrown toenails should start with the proper technique of cutting toenails. This is to cut the toenail straight across with a slight indentation toward the center of the toe. It is also important to make sure that toenails are not too short and that socks and shoes fit properly.

Treatment of an ingrown toenail involves soaking the foot in hot water until the toenail is soft and ready to come off. The next step is to saturate a piece of cotton in an antiseptic and force it under the toenail with the use of a cotton swab, gently lifting the nail away from the flesh.[39] After the toenail is removed, it is important to cover with a sterile dressing to eliminate any possibility of infection. Periodic inspection is important to assure that no complications have arisen due to the loss of the toenail.

TREATMENT OF INJURIES

Treatment of the cause of injury is of vital importance. Treatment of the injury itself will only offer temporary relief. Only be reversing the factors which caused the injury can one hope to prevent recurrences.[40] Because most aerobic training types of injuries result from repetition, the onset and progression of symptoms are of vital importance.

Following are some points of consideration an individual should analyze when an injury has occurred:

1. Progression of current status of pain
2. Pain migration from one location to another location
3. Circumstances surrounding the onset of the injury
4. Proper warm-up
5. Alteration of training routine
6. A significant increase in mileage
7. Defective equipment or shoes
8. Type of terrain training takes place on
9. Past injury problems
10. Structural abnormalities.[41]

To give successful treatment, one should take these points and any other pertinent points into consideration.

Very few injuries related to aerobic training come about suddenly; most injuries give ample advance warning. Most injuries, if treated appropriately at the onset of the first symptoms of pain, can be controlled and chronic problems can be avoided. Not paying attention to early warning signs of potential problems or trying to run an injury out can lead to serious or chronic injuries. Significant changes in eating, drinking, sleeping, or elimination habits can be early symptoms of potential problems.[42]

Another important variable in avoiding injuries is attitude. Setting realistic goals in relationship to training regimen can be very beneficial and vital to the avoidance of unnecessary injuries. Close attention should be paid to signals such as pain, fatigue, or weakness.[43] Aching and tired legs before a training session frequently indicate that the previous training session was too hard.[44] Pushing the body beyond its limits frequently leaves the individual susceptible to injuries and illness. The key to a successful aerobics program is gradualism. An individual does not get out of shape overnight; thus appropriately, one does not get back into shape overnight. A slow, progressive build-up is the most efficient method of training both physically and mentally.

NOTES

[1]Robert M. Parks, "Injuries of the Endurance Athlete," *Medicine Sport,* XII (1978), 140.

[2]John Pagliano, "Pathological Foot Types in Runners," *Medicine Sport,* XII (1978), 165.

[3]Steven Subotnick, "Biomechanics of Running," *Medicine Sport,* XII (1978), 169.

[4]George Sheehan, *Running and Being* (New York: Simon and Schuster, 1978), p. 156.

[5]Subotnick, p. 170.

[6]Parks, p. 152.

[7]Parks, p. 153.

[8]Gerald Mayfield, "Runner's Knee," *Medicine Sport,* XII (1978), 136.

[9]Parks, p. 144.

[10]Parks, p. 146.

[11]Parks, p. 145.

[12]Parks, p. 146.

[13]John P. Curran, *Primer of Sorts Injuries* (Springfield, Ill.: Charles C. Thomas Publishing, 1968), p. 75.

[14]B.J. Brown, *Complete Guide to Prevention and Treatment of Athletic Injuries* (West Nyack, N.Y.: Parker Publishing Co., 1972), p. 189.

[15]Joseph P. Dolan, *Treatment and Prevention of Athletic Injuries* (Danville, Ill.: Interstate Printers and Publishers, 1967), p. 139.

[16]D.Clement, "Tibial Stress Syndrome in Athletes" *Journal of Sports Medicine*, II (1974), 81-85.

[17]Robert Parks, "Injuries of the Endurance Athlete," *Medicine Sport*, XII (1978), 153.

[18]Parks, p. 154.

[19]John Pagliano, "Pathological Foot Types in Runners," *Medicine Sport*, XII (1978), 163.

[20]Pagliano, p. 165.

[21]George A. Sheehan, *Running and Being* (New York: Simon and Schuster, 1978), p. 135.

[22]Pagliano, p. 166.

[23]Pagliano, p. 165.

[24]Robert Buxbaum, *Sports for Life* (Boston: Beacon Press, 1979), p. 70.

[25]John P. Curran, *Primer of Sports Injuries* (Springfield, Ill.: Charles C. Thomas Publishing, 1968), p. 78.

[26]Katherine F. Wells, *Kinesiology*, 6th ed. (Philadelphia: W. B. Saunders Co., 1976), p. 172.

[27]Robert M. Parks, "Injuries of the Endurance Athlete" *Medicine Sport*, XII (1978), 149.

[28]Buxbaum, p. 71.

[29]Charles Bucher, *Fitness for College and Life* (St. Louis: Mosby Publishing, 1985), p. 219.

[30]Parks, p. 150.

[31]Raymond Bridge, *The Runner's Book* (New York: Charles Scribner's & Sons, 1978), p. 151.

[32]Parks, p. 152.

[33]B. J. Brown, *Complete Guide to Prevention and Treatment of Athletic Injuries* (West Nyack, N.Y.: Parker Publishing Co., 1972), p. 26.

[34]Rebecca J. Donatelle, *Access to Health* (Englewood Cliffs, NJ: Prentice Hall, 1988), p. 325.

[35]Joseph R. Dolan, *Treatment and Prevention of Athletic Injuries* (Danville, Ill.: Interstate Printers and Publishers, 1967), p. 95.

[36]Brown, p. 30.

[37]Brown, p. 30.

[38]Brown, p. 37.

[39]Brown, p. 38.

[40]Robert Parks, "Injuries of the Endurance Athlete," *Medicine Sport,* XII (1978), 43.

[41]Parks, p. 143.

[42]Raymond Bridge, *The Runner's Book* (New York: Charles Scribner's Cons, 1978), p. 143.

[43]Robert Buxbaum, *Sports for Life* (Boston: Beacon Press, 1979), p. 64.

[44]Bridge, p. 143.

CROSS TRAINING 13

Cross-training is when you vary and combine different activities as a part of your aerobics program.[1] As mentioned earlier in the text, aerobics is a combination of elevating the pulse rate and increasing the breathing process to continue the activity. Cross-training is an excellent way in which to improve your fitness level and create a little variety in the training program. This type of training has led to many participants looking at training for Triathlon competitions.

BENEFITS OF CROSS-TRAINING

One of the major benefits to cross-training is the fact that it is fun. Most people, to have success in their aerobics program, need to have multiple activities that they can participate in. If the person tries to do just one activity, many times boredom will set in and the person becomes discouraged and will not continue the program. Also, we often find that we lack the facilities necessary to do a certain type of workout or the weather is a challenge that will not allow the person to run outdoors.

Another benefit of cross-training is that it enables a person to maintain their training with less likelihood of injury, staleness, and burnout.[2] As mentioned in the previous chapter, overuse injuries are a major issue with runners. This problem occurs because of the constant pounding the legs take from running on hard surfaces. By doing different aerobic activities you can minimize the possibility of this occurring.

Cross-training is also an excellent way to incorporate the strengthening of different muscle groups. By utilizing different activities in your training program, you can get a more balanced approach toward working all the major muscle groups in the body. Care and thought should be utilized to assure that your training program works on all the major muscle groups.

Another benefit of cross-training is that if you become injured, you should be able to continue to do other types of aerobic activities to maintain your fitness level. Most running injuries involve the lower extremities of the body. If this occurs, activities such as cycling, swimming, water aerobics, and Cross Country Skiing are certainly options that the individual can utilize to maintain high levels of fitness.

EXAMPLES OF CROSS-TRAINING

There are many different ways in which to do cross-training. I would like to concentrate on the three programs of aerobic activities, strength training, and flexibility exercises. The most common aerobic activities participated in would include running, walking, cycling, swimming, rope jumping, cross country skiing, and numerous exercising machines such as Nordic Track, the Gazelle, etc. Any of these activities or any activity that elevates the pulse rate certainly can be an effective way in which to enhance the overall quality of the aerobics program. Another way in which to enhance the quality of a cross-training program is to incorporate a strength training element to your regiment. This can include weight training, calisthenics such as push-ups, etc., and activities such as pull-ups. The goal of a good strength development program should be to work all of the major muscle groups on a regular basis so much thought should be put into the type of training you will be doing. The final component of a good cross-training program should include some type of flexibility component. This should include static and ballistic stretching, yoga, etc.

NOTES

[1] Rosato, Frank, "Fitness for Wellness" 3rd Edition. Minneapolis: West Publishing, 1994.

[2] http://orthoinfo.assoc — reference Cross-Training

APPENDIX A
CHAPTER REVIEWS

CHAPTER ONE

1. Describe the current state of health of adults in our society.

2. Describe the link between a sedentary lifestyle and coronary heart disease.

3. Describe how the theory of calorie consumption and calorie expenditure can result in permanent weight control.

4. Describe the two lifestyle changes that can significantly diminish the on-set of osteoporosis.

CHAPTERS TWO–THREE

1. List three reasons why the 12-minute run–walk test is a good test to be used to assess cardiovascular fitness.

2. What is the easiest and most efficient method of taking the resting pulse rate?

3. How would you determine the minimum heart rate for training during exercising?

4. Describe the method you would use to measure your pulse rate.

CHAPTERS FOUR–SEVEN

1. Describe briefly the three variables needed to be taken into consideration to formulate a successful training program.

2. List and briefly explain three principles that should be followed in starting an aerobics program.

3. Differentiate between a ballistic stretch and a static stretch.

4. Describe two reasons for the necessity of a proper warmup period before the workout.

5. Why is cooling down after a workout so important?

6. Briefly discuss the role that carbohydrates, protein, and fats play in relation to physical performance.

7. How does exercise affect body weight? Food intake?

CHAPTERS EIGHT–NINE

1. Describe three things that change in the heart and circulatory system because of training.

2. Describe three things that change in the respiratory system because of training.

3. Describe three changes to the general body make-up induced by training.

4. Describe two psychological benefits of an aerobics program; sociological benefits.

CHAPTER TEN

1. Describe the proper posture for jogging.

2. Describe the proper foot plant of a jogger.

3. What are the primary limitations of running on your toes?

4. Describe an efficient striding pattern for joggers.

5. Describe the proper use of the arms in jogging.

6. What is the most efficient method of breathing for joggers?

CHAPTER ELEVEN

1. Discuss three considerations in your training that are needed for training in the heat.

2. Describe appropriate clothing for training in the heat.

3. What is the primary cause(s) of heat cramps, heat exhaustion, heat stroke?

4. Discuss three considerations in your training that are needed for training in the cold.

5. Describe the primary differences between training in the heat and the cold.

6. Why is it more difficult to train at higher elevations?

7. Describe the proper mechanics of running hills.

8. Differentiate between training on hard surfaces and soft surfaces.

9. What should you look for when buying a pair of training shoes?

CHAPTER TWELVE

1. Discuss why injuries to runners are characterized as overuse injuries.

2. List three of the more common overuse injuries to runners. Describe preventive techniques for each injury. Describe appropriate treatment for each injury.

3. Discuss why it is so important not to try to "run shin splints out."

4. Describe the proper technique for treating an ankle sprain.

5. Describe the proper technique for treating a blister.

6. Describe some of the key points that need to be analyzed when an injury occurs.

BIBLIOGRAPHY

BOOKS

American College of Sport Medicine. Guidelines for Exercise Testing and prescription. 4th ed., Philadelphia: Lean and Febiger, 1991.

Bogert, L. Jean. *Nutrition and Physical Fitness.* 9th ed. Philadelphia: W. B. Saunders Co., 1973.

Bowerman, William J. *Jogging.* New York: Charter Books, 1967.

Bridge, Raymond. *The Runner's Book.* New York: Charles Scribner's Sons, 1978.

Brown, B. J. *Complete Guide to Prevention and Treatment of Athletic Injuries.* West Nyack, N.Y.: Parker Publishing Co., 1972.

Bucher, Charles. *Fitness for College and Life.* 16th ed., St. Louis: Mosby Publishing, 2007.

- - - - - - - - *Foundations of Physical Education.* 10th ed. St. Louis: C. V. Mosby Co., 19787

Buxbaum, Robert. *Sports for Life.* Boston: Beacon Press, 1979.

Cooper, Kenneth. *The New Aerobics.* New York: M. Evans and Co., 1970.

- - - - - - - - *The Aerobics Way.* New York: M. Evans and Co., 1977.

Corbin, Charles. *Concepts in Physical Education.* 7th ed., Dubuque, Iowa: W. C. Brown Co., 2007.

Costill, David L. *What Research Tells the Coach About Distance Running.* Washington, D. C.: AAHPER Publications, 1968.

Cureton, Thomas K. *Physical Fitness and Dynamic Health.* New York: The Dial Press, 1973.

- - - - -. *Exercise and Fitness.* Chicago: The Athletic Institute, 1969.

Curran, John P. *Primer of Sports Injuries.* Springfield, Ill.: Charles C. Thomas Publishing Co., 1968.

Daniels, Jack. *Conditioning for Distance Running.* New York: John Wiley and Sons, 1978.

deVries, Hubert A. *Physiology of Exercise.* Dubuque, Iowa: W. C. Brown Co., 1980.

Dintiman, George B. *Discovering Lifetime Fitness.* St. Paul, MN: West Publishing, 1984.

Doherty, Kenneth. *Track and Field Omnibook.* 3rd ed. Los Altos, CA.: Track and Field News, 1980.

Dolan, Joseph P. *Treatment and Prevention of Athletic Injuries.* Danville, Ill.: Interstate Printers and Publishers, 1967.

Donatelle, Rebecca J. *Access to Health.* 12th ed., Englewood Cliffs, NJ: Prentice Hall, 2007.

Dyson, Geoffrey, *The Mechanics of Athletics.* 6th ed. London: University of London Press, 1974.

Edington, D. W. *The Biology of Physical Activity.* Boston: Houghton Mifflin Co., 1976.

Falls, Harold B. *Foundations of Conditioning.* New York: Academic Press, 1970.

Fisher, A. Grath. *Jogging.* Dubuque, Iowa: Wm. C. Brown Co., 1980.

- - - - - - -. *Scientific Basis of Athletic Conditioning.* Philadelphia: Lea and Febiger, 1990.

- - - - -. *The Complete Book of Physical Fitness.* Provo, Utah: Brigham Young University Press, 1979.

Fox, Edward. *Sports Physiology.* Philadelphia: W. B. Saunders Co., 1979.

Gabbard, Carl. *Lifelong Motor Development.* Dubuque, Iowa: Wm. C. Brown, Co., 1992.

Garrison, Linda. *Fitness and Figure Control.* 2nd ed. Palo Alto, CA.: Mayfield Publishing Co., 1981.

Getchell, Bud. *Physical Fitness: A Way of Life.* 5th ed., New York: John Wiley & Sons, 2002.

Hoeger, Werner K. *Principles and Labs for Physical Fitness.* 2nd ed., Englewood, CO: Morton Pub., 1990.

- - - - -. *Lifetime Physical Fitness and Wellness.* 3rd ed., Englewood, CO: Morton Pub., 1992.

Jensen, Clayne. *Scientific Basis of Athletic Conditioning.* 3rd ed., Philadelphia: Lea and Febiger Publishing, 1990.

Johnson, Barry L. *Practical Measurements for Evaluation in Physical Education.* 4th ed. Minneapolis, Minnesota: Burgess Publishing Co., 1986.

Kane, William M. Healthy Living: *An Active Approach to Wellness.* Indianapolis, IN: Bobbs-Merrill Pub., 1985.

Krause, Marie V. *Food Nutrition and Diet Therapy.* Philadelphia: W. B. Saunders, 1979.

Levy, D. *The Complete Works of Friedrich Nietzache.* Edinburgh: Foulis Publishing, 1909.

Loy, John W. Jr. *Sport, Culture, and Society.* New York: MacMillan Publishing Co., Inc., 1969.

Luckman, Joan. *Your Health.* Englewood Cliffs, NJ: Prentice Hall, 1990.

Lydiard, Arthur. *Run to the Top.* London: Herbert Jenkins Ltd., 1962.

- - - - -. *Running the Lydiard Way.* Mt. View, Ca.: World Publications Inc., 1978.

Mathews, Donald K. *The Physiological Basis of Physical Education and Athletics.* 4th ed. Philadelphia: W. B. Saunders Co., 1985.

Novich, Max M. *Training and Conditioning of Athletes*. 3rd ed., Philadelphia: Lea and Febiger Publishing Co., 1983.

Pollock, Michael L. *Health and Fitness Through Physical Activity*. New York: John Wiley and Sons, 1978.

Rice, Emmett A. *A Brief History of Physical Education*. New York: The Ronald Press Co., 1958.

Seiger, Lon H. *Walking for Fitness*. 2nd ed., Dubuque, Iowa: W.C. Brown, 1994.

Sharkey, Brian J. *Physiology of Fitness*. Champaign, Ill.: Human Kinetics Publishers, 1979.

Sheehan, George A. *Dr. Sheehan on Running*. 2nd ed., Mt. View, Ca.: World Publications, 1984.

- - - - -. *Running and Being*. New York: Simon and Schuster, 1978.

Updyke, W. F. *Principles of Modern Physical Education, Health and Recreation*. New York: Holt, Rinehart, and Winston Inc., 1970.

Van Aaken, Ernest. *The Van Aaken Method*. Mt. View, Ca.: World Publications, Inc., 1976.

Van Dalen, Deobold B. *The World History of Physical Education*. Englewood, N.J.: Prentice-hall Publishing, 1953.

Wells, Katherine F. *Kinesiology*. 6th ed. Philadelphia: W. B. Saunders Co., 1976.

Williams, Melvin H. *Lifetime Fitness and Wellness*. 2nd ed., Dubuque, Iowa: W.C. Brown, 1994.

Wilmore, Jack H. *Athletic Training and Physical Fitness*. Boston: Allyn and Bacon, Inc., 1977.

PERIODICALS

Astrand, P. O. "Physiological Aspects on Cross-Country Skiing at High Altitudes." *Journal of Sports Medicine and Physical Fitness,* III (1963), 51-52.

Benas, Daphne. "Shin Splints." *Medicine Sport,* XII (1978), 134.

Boyer, J. L "Effects of Chronic Exercise on Cardiovascular Function." *Physical Fitness Research Digest,* II (1972), 1.

Brooks, C.M. "Adult Patricipation in Physical Activities Requiring Moderatre to High Levels of Energy Expenditure." *The Physician and Sports Medicine, XV* (April, 1987), 118.

- - - - -. "Exercise Therapy in Hypertensive Men." *Journal of the American Medical Association,* X (March, 1970), 1668.

Carns, M. L. "Segmental Volume Reduction by Localized verses Generalized Exercise." *Human Biology, XXXII* (1960), 370-376.

Clement, D. "Tibial Stress Syndrome in Athletes." *Journal of Sports Medicine,* II (1974), 81-85.

deVries, Hubert A. "Electromyographic Comparison of Single Doses of Exercise and Meprobromate as the the Effects on Muscular Relaxation." *American Journal of Physical Medicine,* LI (1972), 130-141.

- - - - -. "Prevention of Muscular Distress After Exercise." *Research Quarterly,* XXXII (May, 1961), 177-185.

Doolittle, T. L. "The Twelve-Minute Run-Walk: A Test of Cardiovascular Fitness of Adolescent Boys." *Research Quarterly,* XXXIX (October, 1968), 491-495.

Faria, I. E. "Cardiovascular Response to Exercise as Influenced by Training of Various Intensities." *Research Quarterly,* XLI (March, 1970), 44.

Harris, M. L. "A Factor Analysis of Flexibility." *Research Quarterly,* XL (March, 1969), 62.

Kissen, A. T. "Modification of Thermoregulatory Responses to Cold by Hypnosis." *Journal of Applied Physiology,* XIX (November, 1964), 1043-1050.

Mayfield, Gerald. "Runner's Knee." *Medicine Sport,* XII (1978), 136-138.

McDonald, E.D. "Promoting Active Lifestyles Through Education." *Journal of Physical Education, Recreation, and Dance, 64* (Jan., 1993), 37.

Morgan, W. P. "Psychological Effects of Chronic Physical Activity." *Medicine and Science in Sport,* II (Winter, 1970), 213-218.

Nett, Toni. "Foot Plant in Running." *Track Technique,* XV (March, 1964), 462.

Oscai, L. "Effect of Exercise on Blood Volume." *Journal of Applied Physiology,* XXIV (May, 196), 622-624.

Pagliano, John. "Pathological Foot Types in Runners." *Medicine Sport,* XII (1978), 140-154.

Parks, Robert M. "Injuries of the Endurance Athlete." *Medicine Sport,* XII (1978), 140-154.

Pattengale, P. "Augmentation of Skeletal Muscle Myoglobin by a Program of Treadmill Running." *American Journal of Physiology,* CCSIII (1967), 783-785.

Powell, K.E. "Physical Activity and the Incidence of Coronary Heart Disease." *Annual Review of Public Health, VIII* (1987), 253-287.

Sallis, J.F. "Relation of Cardiovascular Fitness and Physical Activity to Cardiovascular Disease Risk Factors inChildren and Adults." *American Journal of Epidemiology, 127* (1988), 933-941.

Scott, Gladys M. "The Contributions of Physical Activity to Psychological Development." *Research Quarterly,* XXXI (March, 1960), 307.

Shepard, R. J. "What Exercise to Prescribe for the Post-MI Patient." *The Physician and Sports Medicine,* III (January, 1975), 57.

Smith, Everett L. "The Aging process: Benefits of Physical Activity." *Journal of Physical Education, Recreation, and Dance, 57* (Jan., 1986), 33.

Sports Illustrated. "Sports Poll '86." Time Inc., 1986.

Strydom, N. B. "Acclimatization to Humid Heat and the Role of Physical Conditioning." *Journal of Applied Physiology,* XXI (March, 1966), 636-642.

Subotnick, Steven. "Biomechanics of Running." *Medicine Sport,* XII (1978), 169-170.

Surgeon General of the U.S. "Healthy People." U.S. Government Printing Office, 1979.

Taylor, H. L. "The Effect of Sodium Chloride Intake on the Work Performance of Man During Exposure to Dry Heat and Experimental Heat Exhaustion." *American Journal of Physiology,* CXL (1943), 439-451.

U.S. Public health Service. "Healthy People 2000: National Health Promotion and Disease Prevention Objectives." U.S. Government Printing Office, 1990.

Wildavsky, Aaron. "Doing Better and Feeling Worse: The Political Pathology of Health Policy." *Daedalus* (Winter, 1976), 105-123.

Wilmore, Jack. "Body Composition Changes with a 10-Week Program of Jogging." *Medicine and Science in Sports,* II (Fall, 1970), 113-117.

AEROBICS INDEX